I Am Somebody

Telling your story matters

To Nicole

Tamara Faris

By Tamara Faris

Founder of Memory Books for Children
Helping children tell their stories in the midst of loss

I Am Somebody
Telling Your Story Matters

By Tamara Faris
Founder of Memory Books for Children
Helping children tell their stories in the midst of loss

ISBN 978-1-4951-5921-3

www.memorybooks4children.com
PO Box 1372, Gresham, OR 97030

Linda Dodge, Editor & Writing Consultant

Published by Tamara & Ron Faris

July 2015

Contents

Dedicated to helping children
– and adults –
tell their stories in the midst of loss

Foreword

I first met Tamara at her house during an appreciation event that she and her husband, Ron, hosted for the dozens of volunteers who faithfully came each week to create *Memory Books*. I wondered what it was that motivated these people to put in so many hours working on books that would touch children on the other side of the globe. Most of these people had never personally seen the children they were blessing with these *Memory Books*. But they knew Tamara and to know Tamara is to know the vision that God has given her. I'm confident that through reading this book you will come to know Tamara and, more importantly, you will come to know the vision.

Tamara Faris captures the essence of God's call for her global ministry to orphaned children through her book, *I Am Somebody*. During her first visit to South Africa, she encountered orphanages filled with children who had lost ties to any biological family members due to the HIV-AIDs epidemic that ravaged the country's young and middle adult population. God revealed His call to her to return to South Africa to explore the orphans' needs and issues due to their overwhelming suffering. With the blessing of her husband, she left home for an extended time to stay in the orphanages and connect with the children through her warm and loving manner. Through her humble creativity and sensitive grasp of the need for identity in these children, she developed an intervention called the *Memory Book*. The purpose was to address the daunting need to preserve these orphaned children's family stories for their lifetime.

As one of the nursing researchers for the evaluation of the impact of the *Memory Book* intervention, I had the privilege to witness some of the

South African children's first-hand accounts of their precious memories as they paged through their *Memory Books* with us. God showed us how He was using these books to support children's healing from grief, especially when they could share their books with an attentive adult to witness their story of family and origins. During that trip to South Africa, our team visited several of the orphanages and the children's clinic, Sinikithemba, at McCord Hospital where Tamara's outreach to orphaned children originated.

Tamara's faithfulness to implement and extend the *Memory Book* ministry despite challenges and barriers in many parts of the world, including multiple countries in Africa, India, and Haiti, reveals her willingness to answer God's call to serve these children. Tamara relates many stories of God arranging for the volunteers needed to create over 25,000 Memory Books, then shipping these books to remote and often war-torn areas of the world, and His accurate timing and promptings to encourage her and others in His work.

May God use Tamara's heartfelt, sweet stories of discernment and leadership in this effective ministry to orphaned children to help you experience and celebrate the power of God's will for your own life's ministry. May the drama and intrigue of her stories unleash your desire to serve, to listen, and to respond to God's call in your own life, and to see how God fulfills His work throughout the world, one person at a time.

Barb Braband, RN, Ed D
Associate Professor of Nursing
University of Portland, March, 2015

Introduction

Whether you are five or fifty-five, the loss of your mother is something you never get over. Her absence leaves a void that is never filled. When I received the phone call that my mother had died, I felt as if I had been hit by a massive landslide and carried away under the weight of sorrow and grief. I could not breathe. How could it be possible, the woman who had loved and cared for me my entire life was gone? Though I was fifty-five years old, I felt orphaned. Alone. Author Maxine Harris calls it a loss that lasts forever.[1]

As I grapple with my own loss, I cannot help but think about the children around the world who have lost their own mothers as children. How devastating it must be to be a child, orphaned and alone. I think about my own sadness and overwhelming grief and wonder how small children manage to endure through the sadness. I think about what it must feel like for a child to go to bed without the comfort of knowing mother is there, only to wake to the same dreadful reality every single day of their lives.

After the death of my mother, my sister Pamela and I spent months sorting through all of her belongings and distributing them to her seven grandchildren. Lastly, stored away in the basement, we opened a family heirloom trunk to discover artifacts neither of us had ever seen. For hours, the two of us, breathless at times, carefully opened one box after another to find photographs, keepsakes, certificates, and other cherished treasures, many of which had passed from generation to generation.

Hidden deep in the bottom of the trunk, Pamela and I would unearth what would be the most important keepsakes our mother ever preserved.

Photographs of our parents courtship and marriage, of our father, of our family as we were before the divorce and destruction of our family. Pamela and I wept while empty spaces inside us filled with the truth. Our parents loved one another, and their love created us. We were a happy, loving family; and mere children when alcohol, selfishness, and eventual divorce destroyed everything we knew, especially our identities.

Our mother had always spoken of studying her genealogy and writing her story but she never could figure out how to start. She was afraid of computers, and always thought there would be time.

For the next several months, Pamela and I scanned and downloaded the photographs going back generations with names, dates, and captions derived from letters, keepsakes, and other memorabilia to create a photo album called The Hart Kids. We added a family tree going back to an Irishman coming to America aboard a wooden ship, and hardy German stock immigrating through Ellis Island, New York.

All the empty spaces of our childhood began to fill with stories, not told by words, but instead painted by the contents of the trunk. Some stories were clearly told, as in letters and photographs, and others simply by asking. One day Pamela visited a woman our father knew as a teenager. Pamela had remembered this woman's name—a name our mother repelled from when mentioned. Pamela found out our father was her first love, and she still had a bracelet he gave her. She reminisced about how she had married someone else while he was away in the Navy, but had never stopped loving him. The woman said our mother Jean wrote to him while he was deployed, and they were married shortly after he returned home, when she was just seventeen. She gave Pamela a photograph of our father in a reservist uniform, just fifteen himself.

Pamela and I could only surmise about why Mom kept the wedding veil and photographs. To us, this meant our mother never stopped loving our father although they had divorced and she was remarried for thirty-six years. Maybe, the hidden keepsakes deep in the bottom of the trunk represented a part of her story too painful to tell. No wonder she never knew where to start.

But hiding this story left empty spaces in the Hart kids' stories, like the photo albums with which we grew up. My sister and I realized that telling our story matters because our story, like every story, even a painful story, is a part of who we are.

But this sad part of my story would remain just that—sad—if it were to end there. I have discovered that every experience we live, even tragic ones, can be used to write a beautiful and meaningful ending to an otherwise sad life story. Here is my amazing story, I Am Somebody.

Chapter 1

Bedtime Story

April 2005

Fall was approaching in the southern hemisphere. The cool breeze off the Indian Ocean had become warm against the dipping evening temperatures. The huge trees that canopied the estate against the hot daytime temperatures swayed moving the tropical scented warm air up and over the hills and mountains north to the Drakensberg's.

The four-acre estate built by European immigrants to South Africa long ago was full of Dutch Colonial charm. Down the long driveway and through the gates it was as if you had gone back in time to a forgotten lifestyle this home quietly exuded. The two-story sprawling home was designed for an era of sitting rooms, of maids and gardeners, of leisure with tennis court and swimming pool, and of celebration of childhood with exotic pets and an enormous tree house and rope swing.

Today, the contemporary family who lives here rarely uses the sitting room, and chooses to hang out in the converted sunroom with flat screen television and Internet, often eating meals together from the ottoman.

It is nearly eight o'clock and the estate's manicured grounds are dark, except for an outdoor floodlight, a dim light showering the front porch veranda, and a warm light coming from the open kitchen window. The Dutch style half door is typically open to allow evening breezes to cool the house. Tiff, the family pooch, quietly naps outside next to the door.

I had just returned from volunteering as a nurse at a children's village one hour north of here. Danie, the president of an international NGO (non-governmental organization), and his wife Judy had invited me to stay with them off and on during my three months in South Africa. Danie and I were sitting at the kitchen counter visiting about my time at the children's village, waiting for Judy to come home from decorating for her daughter's dance at school.

"Yes! Can you believe it? It was right there under the baby crib!" I half disbelievingly described the event to Danie. "From within my cottage at the children's village I could hear shouting. I went to the open door, peering into the darkness, I asked someone running by what was happening. She said, 'There's a snake coiled up under a baby's crib in House 6!' I followed her to House 6 and pushed past everyone crowded around the doorway. The gardener/security guard had been summoned and there he stood with a bullwhip in his hand. Someone had moved the baby crib away from the wall to reveal one of the deadliest snakes in Africa, a Black Mamba, curled up on top of a child's riding scooter seat. And there in the crib, soundly slept the baby.

"The gardener pushed everyone back away from the doorway to the bedroom, requesting silence. We all held our breath, until we heard a loud crack. Then silence. We didn't know what to think. Then the gardener came from the room, holding the dead snake severed in two. Everyone was shouting and clapping. The whole complex was awake by then. Everyone telling one another what happened. Retelling the story, each time the story growing grander. I went into House 6 to comfort the housemother, and could not believe what I saw: the little baby still asleep in its crib." Danie shook his head with an air of distain. Life in the townships was something he had warned me about, and frankly he had been against my going.

Tiff jumped from the brick back porch barking as she ran toward the car entering the yard. The car's headlights made a swath of light across the yard as Judy turned up the drive and parked right outside the rock wall that circled the pool. Danie looked at his watch.

"Don't worry about dinner," he said as his wife came through the door. "Go up and change, and we will go out to dinner." Danie picked up another cashew from the bowl on the counter and popped it into his mouth. My stomach began to rumble just thinking about dinner. I reached for a cashew.

Judy walked through the dark entryway unhooking one strap of her designer overalls letting it fall. As she climbed the old wooden staircase she stopped, listening as she thought she heard something. Nothing. She reached the long dark hallway, walking past her children's darkened rooms toward the master suite at the end. Again, she stopped. There in the dark, her eyes trying to adjust, she smelled pungent body odor and suddenly sensed the presence of someone near her in the dark. She instantly whirled around and tried to scream, but the air had already escaped from her lungs. Taking another deep breath, Judy let out a wail of wordless desperation.

Flying down the staircase, "Danie!" She screamed, "Danie! Push the panic button!" She screamed again and again, "Push the panic button! There is someone in the house!" Danie immediately hit the alarm button on the kitchen wall above the counter next to the phone and immediately a loud blaring siren filled the air.

Judy came running into the kitchen, shear panic across her face, the strap to her overalls still dangling. I stood frozen to the wall, my heart pounding inside my chest. The sound of crashing and breaking could be heard upstairs while the deafening siren blared out across the neighborhood. Neighbors called. "Yes, there is someone in the house," anxiously reported Danie. I was completely paralyzed with fear. Should I stay here? Or should I try and hide somewhere? It didn't matter either way. I couldn't move. We all stared at one another while the sound of someone's desperate attempt to escape from upstairs continued.

Within minutes, security police vehicles entered the yard and the siren was finally turned off. But the sound of my heart pounding took over in my ears. With guns drawn, the police climbed the wooden staircase and searched every room. "He's gone," they said. "Whoever it was tore the burglar bars away from your daughter's window and escaped across the flat roof over the front porch."

Danie and Judy took inventory and found missing a new laptop he just bought to replace one that had been stolen just weeks before, a DVD player and new amplifier worth $5000. We entered their daughter's room where the heavy steel bars had been torn away from one corner of the window casing with such force it shattered the wood casing and sent wood splinters across the room. Outside the window lying on the roof was a pair of white sneakers.

"It must have been someone who knew where the things were," shouted an angry Danie. Having recently hired someone to do remodeling in the house, Danie reviewed all the places that could have been surveyed while someone worked on the property. The bushes along a long, dark driveway could easily hide someone waiting to enter behind one of our cars before the gate closed. The five-foot high security wall only spans the front portion of the property. The old wire fencing across the back could be jumped by nearly anyone.

"That's it," yelled Danie. "That's the third break in within the last few months. We are no longer safe in this house."

"But this is our family home," Judy sobbed.

Danie arranged for the security police to stay during the night, and then he planned to make arrangements the next day for permanent 24-hour security.

"Tamara, we don't want you to sleep alone in the guest wing tonight," said Judy. She and I walked through the scullery that separated the guest wing and my room from the main house. I gathered up some clothes, my laptop, phone, and some toiletries. "You can sleep in an extra room next to ours tonight. Fortunately, our daughter is spending the night with a friend. That will give us time to repair her room. I don't want her to see the damage done to the window bars."

Judy opened the door to an extra bedroom at the end of the hall next to theirs. Inside were twin antique beds piled high with handmade quilts. Across the room was a stately old wooden armoire. The room appeared to be the final resting place for sentimental heirlooms that no longer suited a more cosmopolitan décor. Judy pulled the white linen curtains closed.

"We're right next-door. I am so sorry. Please don't worry," she said as she reached out to offer a reassuring hug. Then she closed the door and left me alone.

With adrenalin still coursing through my body and my heart pounding irregularly inside my chest, I had no idea how I would sleep. Forgoing my typical bedtime ritual of a hot bath, I put on pajamas and slid under the heavy bedding in the darkened room. I felt like the frightened child I was when I slept overnight at my grandparents' home when my parents were away. Warm tears ran from the corners of my eyes and down into my ears as I longed to be held by someone safe. I could not stop looking at the white curtains covering the windows lit by the outdoor floodlight. My mind raced with the fear of someone climbing to the flat roof outside, the shadow of his or her form etched on the linen fabric. Would they be holding a hatchet? I imagined. Would they slowly open the window and somehow climb through the burglar bars and enter the room? Maybe if I hide under the blanket they wouldn't see me in the dark. I closed my eyes.

I reached out for my phone on the bedside table, and entered the long distance number for home.

"Hi, Donna, is Ron in?"

"Oh hi, Tamara. Yes, I will get him for you," she replied.

I practiced speaking with a calm voice as I waited for him.

"Tamara?" came a familiar voice.

Deep within me came an uncontrollable sob. "Oh, honey, I'm okay. Please don't be worried. Something awful happened here tonight," my voiced interrupted while I tried to breathe.

"Are you okay?" questioned Ron.

"I will be. Danie and I were waiting for Judy to come home from her daughter's school where she had been decorating. She went upstairs to get changed for dinner and found a robber was in the house. She is okay. We are all okay. But, it was just so scary. I have never been so frightened in my life. Judy came screaming downstairs when she realized someone was hiding in the dark hallway. Honey, it is just so frightening to think about what could have happened to her."

Ron was quiet. "By the time the police came, he and whoever else might have been helping him had somehow gotten away. Oh, honey, I feel like I am having a heart attack. My heart is pounding so hard. It's just so frightening to be here. I've been told it's a federal offense to steal from a house when the homeowners are home. It means prison if you are caught. They'd rather hack you to death than go to prison. Oh, honey, I'm so sorry to worry you. Please don't worry about me. Danie has arranged for security guards tonight, and then he is going to arrange for 24-hour security. He is really upset because they can't seem to keep people from breaking into their house. I think he's really worried that something awful is going to happen. Some friends had an intruder come into their bedroom while they slept. The intruder beat the husband and held the family hostage while others ransacked the house. They have young girls who are so frightened they can't return to their home."

I stopped when I realized I probably had said too much. "I miss you. I wish I was with you right now."

"I miss you too, darling," Ron quietly assured me. "Lets talk tomorrow. Try and sleep. I will pray you will sleep. I love you."

"I love you too, darling."

In the darkness of the room, my heart began to calm and I listened over and over again in my mind to the sound of Ron's voice. Like a lullaby, his words are comforting and assuring, "Let's talk tomorrow." I sank into a deep sleep.

Chapter 2

Below the Fold

October 2004 - six months earlier

"Well, how long were you thinking?" Ron asked while sipping his coffee.

"I can get a visa for three months without any problem. Dr. Holst said I could stay at the doctors' quarters at the hospital and either work at the hospital or at Sinikithemba. I just keep thinking about what she said."

"What's that?" Ron questioned.

"Remember after the hospital tour when she and I were in the hallway? She put her hand on my arm and, with tears welling up in her eyes, said, 'Tamara, my greatest fear is that while the world is focused on the next natural disaster, a whole continent of people will disappear.' The whole world rightfully mourns as 250,000 people died in the Indonesian tsunami in a matter of moments. But 250,000 people die of AIDS every month in Africa and it is no longer front-page news. It's a tired topic, like someone with a chronic illness that people get tired of hearing about.

"You probably won't be able to stop thinking about what we saw there last spring. Remember the precious little girl in the green sweater? She, along with dozens of other children orphaned by AIDS came to a place where she could stay during the day and eat. The women would cook enough rice and beans at lunch so they could fill small containers to send with the children to eat at night. Then most of them simply lie on the floor in someone's home to sleep at night.

"Dr. Holst said I should consider coming back and volunteering as a nurse, and that way I would at least feel like I have done something.

I knew when I read Dr. Holst's email that I was going to go. I know it sounds crazy, but I think I am going to South Africa and volunteer as nurse. I just need you to be onboard 100%. I'll need your help with Mom while I'm gone and I'll need you to help convince the kids their mom hasn't gone off the deep end. I know they'll think this is crazy. I think this is crazy. But I know inside I'm supposed to go."

Six months later

I have done everything I thought would prepare me to be away in South Africa for three months. I went to the local library and left with a stack of books I cleared from the South Africa shelf. I began to read one after another. The Boer War, history of the Zulu Tribe, and wars with the Dutch and English, apartheid, the imprisonment and eventual presidency of Nelson Mandela, the future of the government led by the majority African National Congress, and Bishop Desmond Tutu's "No Future Without Forgiveness." I read novels describing the awful years of apartheid and look through photo albums made by photographers recording the lives of those left behind by AIDS.

I cleared my own library shelves of books I had acquired over the years while I trained in child grief and loss and volunteered with a local organization that helps children living with loss. Since I am a care-giver for my mom, I arranged for family and friends to provide her additional help. I even purchased birthday gifts, signed Easter cards, and arranged them on the counter so Ron could deliver them. All in an effort to make my absence less noticeable or painful for those I will leave behind. I know I am deluding myself to think I can simply leave my life without a ripple of effect on the lives that intersect mine.

Without doubt, however, the most important thing I have done is to spend time in prayer and devotion each day. While previously I may have quickly read a passage from my favorite devotional, I now spent at least one hour each morning in quiet reflection.

To be honest, I am scared to death to leave home alone. During my marriage, the longest I had been away from Ron was one week while I volunteered as a nurse for a foster kids summer camp. There have been times in the last few weeks that I've wondered if there was any way I could graciously get out of going. From the moment I said yes, I began to doubt and secretly regret it.

Frankly, the decision to go to South Africa and volunteer as a nurse for three months came over me and I simply said yes. Then came the thoughts of missing my husband, my family, my bed, my clothes, my favorite restaurant, my stuff. I hate to admit that while the "brave and courageous decision to go to Africa" makes me look like an amazingly selfless person, honestly, inside I am quite selfish. The choices I've made in the past to do good things publicly have always taken into consideration, the convenience, the comfort, the conditions, and even the compensation.

Once while traveling to Spain on a mission-type trip, my two large suitcases bulging with enough clothes and toiletries to fill an entire boutique didn't arrive—to my horror. A friend took pity on my pathetic situation and loaned me something to wear. When my luggage arrived I had to lug it uphill through cobblestone streets, up five flights of stairs, and also endure the heartless laughter of everyone when I had to admit nothing I packed belonged on a mission trip, including my cherished pink sequined sweater!

I don't dare think about actually getting on a plane and flying halfway around the world and being away for three months. Daily I dwell on my faith and my family, and hope I can convince God to go with me.

The family is all assembled for a going away party. My bags are packed and my flight leaves at 11 p.m. tonight. For two days, I've had butterflies in my stomach and secretly hope I am coming down with a dreadful illness that will not permit me to board a plane. But I am too proud to admit I am truly scared to death when everyone is so excited for what I am about to do: travel to Africa to save the world.

I unwrap a beautiful handmade journal with photos of every member of my family, with jewels and ribbons, with the words HOME, treasure, Ron loves Tamara, and Africa 2005 covering the front and inside. My sister Pamela writes on the first page, "When you need us most while you are away, I hope you find comfort from our smiling faces," Written below a bird with an olive branch in its beak: Use your wings and fly!

As the plane lifts into the dark skies and the twinkling lights of my hometown disappeared, I hold close to my chest a large envelop of letters from those I love, and I cry. I know nothing about this journey, except for one thing. I feel the presence of God with me. And somehow that is enough.

Chapter 3

A Reflection

After a grueling 32-hour flight and a weekend rest at Danie and Judy's home they call Meryckton, Judy drives me the half hour to McCord Hospital located near downtown Durban. I meet Geraldine who would give me an orientation tour of the hospital and clinics, and then help me settle into my room at the resident doctor's quarters. The first thing she did was to hand me my name badge, and then she chastised me for coming so late in the day. Geraldine may only be a subordinate here, but I could tell she was someone with a lot of power. Experience taught me she was someone to have in my corner.

I turn my name badge over and there in bold letters is who I would be known as for the next three months: Visitor. Something inside tells me I will have to earn a title here, a million miles from the personal and professional accolades I've rested on.

The hospital complex includes a four-story hospital, a social and psychology clinic, an HIV/AIDS clinic, teaching, research, and administration offices, and a cafeteria and housekeeping building spread over several blocks straddling a hilly terrain overlooking downtown Durban in Kwa Zulu Natal, the birthplace of the Zulu people. At city's edge lies the warm water of the Indian Ocean extending to the horizon and beyond.

After a tour, wet with sweat from the heat and tropical humidity, and still jet-lagged, Judy and Geraldine help me carry my book-filled luggage downstairs into the basement of the Doctor's Quarters, my home for the next 3 months. It reminded me of a college dorm room with a twin bed, nightstand, desk with wooden chair, a built-in closet and vanity, and one overhead light. Geraldine hands me two keys, one for the outside door, and one for my room.

"The outside door is locked at all times. There is a nighttime security guard at the door. Keep your room locked at all times, even when you are here. Sinikithemba HIV/AIDS Clinic starts at 7:30 a.m. "They're expecting you," Geraldine instructs with a stern voice and a smile.

I close the door behind them and turn the key, and suddenly a wave of sadness hits me. I swallow, and the lump in my throat painfully cuts as it travels into my chest. Never in my life have I ever felt so uncertain about what lays before me. I have never felt so alone.

I unpack and hang the few clothes I brought in the closet, arrange my toiletries on the vanity. I carefully tape some drawings made by my grandkids to the mirror and set photos and my alarm clock by the bed. I unlock my door and walk the few steps to the basement kitchen where I find an empty cupboard I can store the few groceries I purchased with Judy. I set up my laptop and phone charger on the desk and plug the adaptor into the wall outlet. As I plug the charger cord into my computer, a large spark flies from the outlet, and the overhead light goes out.

Great. I probably blew a circuit. I walk down the hall and can't find any circuit panel. The place is quiet with no one to ask. I go back to the room and decide I would deal with the disappointment by trying to act as if nothing had happened. I had planned to continue my running routine while in South Africa. I lace up my running shoes and lock the door behind me.

I run down the street between hospital and clinics and onto the main thoroughfare where I had traveled with Judy earlier that day. I run for about fifteen minutes then I turn again down another street heading down toward the ocean for another fifteen minutes. Retracing my steps, I return back up the hill to the Doctor's Quarters and meet two women wearing white lab coats in the stairwell.

"Went for a run?" one of them asks.

"Yes," I responded, upbeat.

"Oh, never do that alone. Next time you want to go for a run, I can go with you," offered one of the women, as neither one slowed to continue our conversation.

"Oh, that would be great," I hollered as they went out of sight. "Hey!" I yell, wanting to ask them about the circuit breaker. They are already gone.

I shower and notice there was no lock on the community bathroom/ shower door directly across the hall from my room. The thought of a leisure shower evaporates.

I go into the kitchen and make a small bowl of yogurt mixed with muesli, a handful of almonds, and boiled water for a cup of African rooibos tea. Next to the kitchen is a large meeting room with sofas and a television. Still quiet.

I walk into my room and lock the door behind me. The sun had set and my room is dark. I stand on my bed in an attempt to see out the window, but can only see razor wire across the top of a fence. I sit down on the end of my bed in the dark, and unexpectedly feel tears well up in my eyes.

I feel so alone. What am I doing here? Here in this basement room, without even a view outside. Then I catch my reflection in the dimly lit mirror over the vanity.

Tamara? A quiet familiar voice crosses my mind. It sounds like my voice, but always says things that are simple yet truly profound. *I didn't bring you to Africa because of my love for the people here, but because of my love for you.* It was at this moment, I begin to realize coming here was about something more than anything I was going to do here for the people of Africa.

I feel naked sitting there before the mirror. All I can see was what I am feeling. There are no fancy clothes or expensive jewelry to hide behind. No manmade image created by prideful public accomplishments. There is nothing but a small face looking through the dark back at me. Is that really me? I quietly thought.

Tamara? This is the only view you'll need from this room. Right here in this mirror.

Chapter 4

Author Unknown

Though it is only 7:30 in the morning, the air is already warm and humid. Dressed in my nursing scrubs, my white time-tested nursing shoes, and my Visitor name badge, I hike the short distance from the Doctor's Quarters to Sinikithemba (sin-a-ka-tem-ba) HIV/AIDS Clinic. I have been awake since 1 am, and this moment could not come soon enough. This is my first day on the job volunteering as a nurse in Africa.

Butterflies of anxiety swirl inside my stomach. Perspiration beads gather on my brow, and against my back beneath my backpack filled with nursing equipment, my journal, and a water bottle. Hidden from view, I wear a money belt filled with American dollars and South African rand equaling $3000. Every penny I brought to live on.

Security police dress in bright yellow shirts and black pants and line the street dissecting the hospital complex. Their presence and smiles were a welcomed relief for me knowing it is risky carrying so much money, but a greater risk leaving it in my room. The decision of carrying all that money at all times felt silly and smart all at once.

As I pass through the guarded security gate, I think for a minute I hear beautiful singing coming from inside the two-story white building. I stepped through the back door and took a seat inside the reception room filled with people, yes, singing. I looked around the room and recognized clinic staff I had met during my orientation. I quietly closed my eyes and listened. The tune was familiar, yet the language was not. Could it be, though I have traveled 10,000 miles from home God, indeed, is in this place?

I smile as I remember reading from Psalms: "If I rise on the wings of the dawn, if I settle on the far side of the sea, even there your hand will guide me, your right hand will hold me fast." (Psalm 139:9-10 NIV)

Without a moment to catch my breath, I am swept away with a team of physicians who are going to an AIDS center twenty minutes away. It appears my reputation has preceded my arrival when Dr. Henry Sunpath erroneously introduces me as a cancer specialist. Working as a nurse on an oncology unit is far from being a cancer specialist in America; however, here in this place where thousands of people die everyday of AIDS, help and hope is sought anywhere. I thought it would be an introduction difficult to live up to, but felt confident I wouldn't need to defend it my first day.

As I followed close behind, Dr. Arbuckle, head physician of the Dream Centre, begins to tell me about a young man upstairs who is suffering the ravages of testicular cancer literally eating away at his body. With treatment limited to palliative (comfort) care, I wondered if anything in my nursing arsenal would provide a strategy equal to a miracle this man surely needed.

Before we even reach the doorway of his room the odor of dying flesh filled my nostrils. Two nurses tending to the man immediately covered him, their eyes searching mine as they quietly leave. Dr. Arbuckle introduces the patient to me, explaining his diagnosis of cancer due to compromised immune system or AIDS as he lifted the white sheet covering his torso. My mind fills with nursing techniques for comfort and cleanliness; pain management, debridement of the wound seem primary to his care. But as Dr. Arbuckle covers him, I look into the man's eyes and realize compassion is this man's greatest need.

As the physicians continue their rounds I cannot help but think of the nurses working here in this place. Sisters, they are called here in South Africa, fully educated and skilled to do this work. The Dream Centre appeared to be adequately staffed. Then why would I need to be in this place? It felt as if I would be stepping in the way of another nurse, taking her job that she is here to do.

Tamara? I hear the still quiet voice again inside my head. *What's needed is someone who has the time to offer an abundance of compassion. Someone who can sit and listen to someone's story, his or her heartache or dream, someone skilled in helping those suffering from loss and grief.*

After an exhausting day, I return to my room in the doctor's quarters. I bathe and eat a handful of almonds, a sliced mango and hot tea. Lying in the dark I watch as horizontal pulses of lightning race across the sky crackling with an occasional boom.

I lie in silence while voices in my head repeat the diagnoses and prognoses of men and women battling disease like a tsunami sweeping across this land, taking with it thousands upon thousands of lives everyday. Leaving in its wake no one untouched by loss and grief.

Even a tiny infant recognizes the absence of his mother's scent while he suckles when AIDS takes her away. When the arms that hold are not hers, even an infant grieves. Small children wonder why a mother whom they love would leave them all alone. Though young themselves, children are caring for children when no one else is there. No one would know that behind a child's smiling face is a story of loss, a loss that lingers forever.

For every man and woman I met today, there are those they love who will be left behind when their lives ebb quietly to an end. Sons and daughters, mothers and fathers, families forever changed when someone they love dies of AIDS.

Dr. Sunpath asked if I will plan to come again to the Dream Centre. Lying still in my bed, I ask myself, will I come? Will I volunteer to come where no one volunteers to go? Will I abandon why I think I came, and simply go?

Each morning during the first week in South Africa, I ride to the Dream Centre with Dr. Sunpath and doctors doing their residency at McCord Hospital who conduct rounds and update care plans for patients. Initially I join them, but often choose to stay behind with a patient with whom I want to talk.

Usually my interest in staying is met with suspicion by the patient, but often melts away with stories about loved ones or their fears, or hopes and dreams. One young man tells me all he wants to do is make his son smile. A woman sharing a room with three other women looks outside her window to the rolling green hills below and wonders if she will ever feel grass beneath her feet again.

After missing my ride back to the doctor's quarters one day, I am waiting outside the Dream Centre for a hospital shuttle to come for me. A small red pick-up truck enters through the security gate and backs up to the door. Several young men sit on the edge of the truck bed, and lying at their feet is a small frail body in a dress. A few strands of hair cover her head; her limbs are thin and contorted.

I think to myself, oh poor soul, she didn't make it in time. She has already died. The young men open the tailgate of the truck, apparently not knowing where else to take their dead relative. As they begin to move her, she begins to wail and writhe. I jump, startled to learn this young girl was not a corpse but alive. The next day I find her propped up in bed eating a cheese sandwich and making her roommates laugh by telling stories about the rumor of her demise when she arrived.

Following rounds one day, I return to a woman's bedside where earlier that day the attending doctor had told the nurses she was actively dying. With multiple diagnoses of diseases, many that would kill you by themselves, AIDS had left her body unable to defend against tuberculosis, cancer and hepatitis C. Often times the treatment of diseases cannot be administered simultaneously with anti-retro-viral drugs, so it becomes a choice between continuing to treat HIV and allowing other diseases to manifest themselves. Or treat the disease while allowing the viral load of HIV in the blood stream to increase unabated; the choice only that of the better of two evils.

I move a chair from the corner of the room and sit near the bedside. She lay as though in death's repose, yet on close inspection I can see her chest rise and fall with shallow breath. I place my hand upon her hand and wonder if she knows I am there.

In my mind I ask, Are you someone's mother? Or daughter? Or sister? Do they know how sick you are? Will they arrive here in time to say good-bye? Or have they already left you behind when they too have died? Oh, how sad to be alone when you are dying, I thought. Then it came to me, she wasn't alone. I am there with her. Not because I had to be, but because I choose to be. I hear someone come into the room, but they quickly leave before I can even turn to see who it is.

I wish you could tell me who you are, I thought to myself. I whisper under my breath, do you know how much God loves you? Her chest continues to rise and fall.

Death may seem very foreign, even frightening to most. But as a nurse I have had many of my patients die. I have witnessed many people saying good-bye to someone they love. I have seen children standing at the end of a bed, or against the wall outside the door, when someone they love has died; I am left wondering how this will affect their lives.

Early in my nursing career after the death of a patient, I had to find a perspective about dying so I could continue to nurse. Whether a birth or dying, humans only experience it once. I consider it an honor to be present for either. Though death ends the physical life, most people's lives will continue to impact others even after they have died through memories and shared experiences. Death may leave a gaping hole in someone's life, but remembering the life you shared can help fill the emptiness.

Absent the late afternoon sun, the room has cooled with dark evening shadows. My heart grieves because I know I must leave soon, yet I sense death is close for this young woman. Her skin is cool and rigid. The heartbeat and breath are interrupted by moments of none.

I take my hand away from hers, and wonder if she is pleading inside for me to stay. I know there is a part of this journey she must make on her own. I quietly wonder, Is this what is called the valley of the shadow of death? The space between life and death where one must let go of the hand of those they love and walk ahead alone?

I begin to recite the 23rd Psalm in my mind. *The Lord is my shepherd; I shall not want. He maketh me to lie down in green pastures; he leadeth me beside the still waters. He restoreth my soul: he leads me in the paths of righteousness for his name's sake. Yea, though I walk through the valley of the shadow of death, I will fear no evil; for thou art with me; they rod and thy staff they comfort me. Thou preparest a table before me in the presence of mine enemies; thou anointest my head with oil; my cup runneth over. Surely goodness and mercy shall follow me all the days of my life; and I will dwell in the house of the Lord forever.*

Chapter 5

A Graphic Illustration

It is Friday evening following my first week in South Africa. I am waiting outside the doctor's quarters on the corner near the Nursing School dorm. Judy called earlier in the week with an invitation to stay at Meryckton with her friends while Danie travels to the United States for meetings. My backpack is filled with computer and camera, books and my journal, and my money belt. At my feet lay my smaller luggage jammed with nearly every piece of clothing I brought, which is now in need of cleaning.

My rented cell phone rings. It is my son, Joshua, on his way home from the nightshift as a police officer. The weight of my workweek lifts as we talk to one another. It is our first contact since leaving eight days ago so neither of us wants to hang up. "I love you honey." "I love you too, Mom. Jenny sends her love. Be safe."

"I just couldn't stand the idea of you spending the entire weekend alone at the hospital," Judy said as the car zoomed up the N3 freeway toward Hilcrest. The N3 begins in Durban teeing off the major north/south N2 that takes you north to Richards Bay and Mozambique or south to Port Elizabeth and further to Cape Town. An hour north on the N3 is Pietermaritzburg and eventually leads to Johannesburg, considered one of the most dangerous cities in the world.

Pulling into the long driveway, I am amazed at how beautiful and green the landscape is after a week in a city of cement. Tiff runs out to greet the car and welcome me home. Angie, the housekeeper, shyly smiles as I pull my luggage through the kitchen on my way to the guest wing. "Sawbona (hello)," she quietly says. "Sawbona Ang," I reply slowing to smile.

The guest room is as I left it. The white iron double bed holds mountains of pillows and a white cotton duvet coverlet. The full-length window is framed with beige drapes. I open the window to a cool breeze and the sound of the guinea hens pecking through the grass.

I immediately fill the large pink porcelain tub and slide into the hot water, letting the water continue to flow. I feel like a child, unable to reach the end with my toes; I simply float while completely submerged. I wish I could stay here forever, I think, as I close my eyes and drift to a peaceful place. Only He knows what a tub of my favorite color—pink—would mean to me. In small ways, God shows me how much He loves me. In this moment I realize we can never out-give Him.

My mind wanders. How can it be that two completely different worlds can share the same space? History tells, not very well. From the beginning of civilization, tribal wars among Zulu and Xhosa dominated for land, followed by wars between immigrating white Europeans to gain possession of the vital link between Europe and The Far East. In 1652, the Dutch East India Company founded a shipping station at the Cape of Good Hope, but lost its hold to the British government in 1806, when England took permanent possession of South Africa. This important link to England's greatest oversees possession, India provided opportunity to ferry desirable goods from the Far East back to the upper crust of citizenry, and to exploit the land and the hidden treasures beneath its soil.[2]

Haaaa! Haaaa! I jump from my near slumber to the sound of the obnoxious Haddidah (ha-de-dah) bird somewhere in the yard. Haaaa! Haaaa! I hear Tiff run by the window barking as another Haddidah protests, Haaaa! Haaaa!

Beneath the warm water, I feel hidden from the concerns I have faced all week and wish I could forget. But how do you forget the faces of those who are fighting the greatest battle this country has ever encountered: HIV/AIDS.

All week hundreds of men, women and children, often very ill, travel by public transportation or by foot, line up at the doorway of Sinikithemba (means place of hope) HIV/AIDS Clinic with hope of qualifying for anti-retro-viral medication. The clinic reception room chairs fill signaling all that the clinic can see each day. Many who had traveled great distances are turned away by staff, but encouraged to return again.

Across this beautiful land, its greatest resource is disappearing by entire generations, succumbing to a foe that will kill more people than any war this country has ever fought. Without consideration for skin color, social status, age, or gender, HIV/AIDS has infected millions of people, and will have orphaned 2.2 million South African children by 2015.[3] Even newborn babies are assaulted by the diagnosis before they take their first breath. Dr. Holst's words echo in my mind, "An entire continent of people may disappear."

Judy and her friends have set the outdoor table with fine linen and white dishes. The table is covered with trays of beautifully prepared herb chicken and roasted vegetables. Fresh fruit, figs, cheeses, olives are neatly arranged. Homemade warm bread straight from the oven is thinly sliced and covered with a linen napkin. At the end of the table is a full tea service, including clotted cream, brown sugar crystals, and honey. A tin holds black tea and African rooibos.

Amidst the laughter of friends, I quietly allow every morsel of food to linger in my mouth as though it were the first time eating such delicacies. I sit back and sip on a hot cup of rooibos and wonder if these women know anything about what I have seen this week. Though their lives are certainly not without pain, do they know what it is like when fellow South Africans are losing everyone they love? What would it be like if each one of these friends died one after another until there was no one left?

The sun has set and the air has cooled. Judy returns from the kitchen with a warm pudding (cake covered with vanilla pudding) dolloped whipped crème and vanilla ice cream. Oh, I wish I could stay here forever, I think to myself. I quietly realize that not even I want to think about the battle that is being waged outside these walls. Not tonight at least.

CRACK! I hear a loud crack, but do not know what it is. Suddenly I realize I am on the floor of the scullery. And there is blood across my lap. For a moment, I am stunned. Judy rushes to my side, "Oh, Tamara!" My head is throbbing. Blood begins to drip from my chin. "Oh, Tamara! You've fallen and hit the cabinet. You've split your forehead open." I pull back my bloody hand from my forehead. Slowly everything is starting to make sense. While bringing dishes into the scullery, I slipped on the wet terracotta tiles and hit my head on a corner of the wood cabinet. The crack I heard was my forehead hitting the sharp wooden corner of a cabinet.

Holding a cold cloth to my forehead, Judy and a friend help me to my feet. Upon inspection I realize the one-inch gapping gash beneath the eyebrow of my left eye is deep enough it needs stitches. But South Africa is the last place I want someone to use a needle on me. Though a nurse, I have witnessed but never stitched a wound closed.

Judy and I drive to the all night pharmacy and they let me through the locked door once they see my face. After the pharmacist agrees I need stitches, he reluctantly puts together a small suture kit with steri-strips, 2 X 2 sterile gauze, tape, and antibiotic crème, and then briefly gave me a tutorial.

An ice pack has slowed the bleeding, and numbed my forehead. Without knowing how I am going to do this, I reject the help of others and close the door of a hallway powder room. Feeling the wound sufficiently cleaned by all the bleeding, I organize all the supplies inside the sink. The small mirror in the dimly lit room must do. The wound is blanched white due to both the trauma and the ice. The crack I heard when I fell was the bone over my left eye hitting the wood in one grand smack quick and clean, leaving a straight cut.

Following the pharmacist's directions, I use the small circular needle and thread and attempt to insert the needle through the lower flap of skin; a wave of nausea overwhelms me and I feel faint. Holding the sink I take a few deep breaths. Placing the needle back in its package, I decide instead to attach stereo-strips to the lower center of the gash and lift the skin to meet the other side a half dozen times. Stitches would have allowed me to get the wound wet, but now I'll have to keep it dry for a couple weeks. It actually looks pretty good. After antibiotic crème, I bandage it with sterile gauze and tape and then present myself to a horrified audience outside the door.

Bidding Judy and friends goodnight, I go to the guest room where I discover a large black eye forming and an oppressive headache. Sliding into bed I think about all the scars I see on the faces of South Africans. Some scars are the result of Zulu tribal customs, but many left simply by the ravages of African life.

Initially I fear what my patients will think when they see my black eye and swollen eyebrow, but I would later realize when they look into my eyes, their eyes tell me I now know first hand the ravages that define their lives.

Chapter 6

No Fairytale Ending

One week after another pass quickly by. Weekdays fill with activities such as conducting adherence training for patients recently beginning an ARV regimen at Sinikithemba. If patients miss follow-up appointments for more than two months, their names are removed from the anti-retro viral treatment, and they must go to the back of the line again. Adherence is vital for success of drug treatment, yet the stigma of infection often keeps people from following through with treatment when they must explain the need to miss work, school, or must simply be home with family. I have an opportunity to assist a physician with education of newly pregnant women who are HIV positive. Early research shows HIV positive transmission rates during birth are reduced from 79% to 4% among women who choose to give birth by caesarean section.[4]

Sinikithemba has a children's play area outside the building under a porch overhang. Two young women volunteer to entertain the children while they wait for the appointment for either their relative or they themselves. When time permits, I join them on the porch. Without describing the concept, I practice reflective play and reflective art with the children while the volunteers watch. A young child sits at a child-size table with paper and crayons. She lays her head on her paper hiding her work from me. When she reaches for another color crayon I simply say the color. Time and time again, I respond to her choices of color by stating what exactly she had chosen. As she colors, she slowly begins to lift her head from her drawing, revealing it to me. She begins to respond to me by choosing different colors faster and faster. Eventually we are both laughing. In the end, she is proud to show me her work. She has discovered she can create something beautiful that gives her joy, even if only momentarily.

Each morning I leave the doctor's quarters, I look at the pile of books and manuals I brought with the hope I will find someone or some place here at McCord Hospital or Sinikithemba to share about the impact of loss on a child and the unresolved grief that lingers frozen inside, often for a lifetime.

One evening a physician completing her residency at McCord asks if I want to go with her to house sit while a South African physician is away. While sitting in the window of this magnificent home watching a lightning storm across the Indian Ocean, she tells me her life story. Shortly after her mother became pregnant with her, her father died in an auto accident. She grew up never knowing the man who would have been her father, and unknowingly has grieved a man she never knew.

I explain that when loss occurs, we grieve the empty space that person holds in our life. Even after the outward mourning of that loss ends, a universal human response called grieving continues internally for a lifetime. As with a father, or a mother, it is a loss that is forever because no one can ever replace them. Externally we attempt to convey we are over the pain of losing someone important to us, but internally symptoms often rarely associated with loss invade every aspect of our lives. Anger and depression are often the result of loss. Sleeplessness, headaches, stomachaches, poor concentration, and broken relationships may result because grief lies deep and unresolved.

When children lose someone dear to them, like a mother or father, it often times can lead to paralysis of developmental phases, such as trust, autonomy, industry, and independence.[5] The inability to trust or crippling fear can be the result of loss experienced as a child. Alan Wolfelt says, "If a child is old enough to love he is old enough to grieve."[6]

Tears glisten on her face as lightning lights the room that has become dark. "It all makes so much sense," she said. "Every relationship I have ever had has failed. I simply have not been able to trust anyone with my heart."

One day I ask Onnie (Oh-knee), the housekeeper for the doctor's quarters, to place on the physician's bed a book by Donna Schuurman, *Never the Same*.[6] Schuurman writes of her own childhood loss, the impact of grief and loss, and ways to foster healing after losing someone dear. Later that week, I find the book returned on my bed with a note that reads: *If this information is what you came to South Africa to do, don't leave until you've told someone. This book has changed my life.*

Chapter 7

Pages of My Heart

After weeks in Africa, I spend late evening hours and early morning hours writing about the day's events. My thoughts and feelings fill the pages of the journal, much like talking with a trusted friend. During the many hours alone, I lie on my bed and read and reread the pages of the journal as though I am reading the story of someone I do not know. I am often times taken back by what I am reading. But this is not someone else's story. This is my story. I am living this life—a life no longer constrained by self-imposed limitations that has previously dictated my entire life.

For the first time in my life, I sense my true self emerging from deep within. No longer hiding behind the vestiges of a pampered external life, whom I truly am inside is free to come alive. The frightened child inside has learned that my fear can be overcome, that my shame that created a person in need of doing instead of simply being me.

When I arrived weeks ago, my greatest fear was the time I was locked alone inside my room. I had cultivated a life that appears to be perfect from all other vantage points except the one that is most important: from within. I have discovered in this place a fondness for the face looking back at me from the vanity mirror of my room.

While at Sinikithemba, I continue to look for opportunities to share what I know about child grief and loss with anyone who will listen. A Sinikithemba staff person tells me that prior to my coming, a graduate student from England was working on similar work with children. She had spent much of her time in South Africa living at an orphanage called Lily of the Valley. She suggests I contact the woman who manages the orphanage and request a visit.

With only one month left before I return home, I convince Marion at Lily of the Valley to allow me to visit for two weeks. She was hesitant at first, being skeptical there was anything I could accomplish inside of two weeks, as most volunteers coming to Lily commit to one year of service. I arrange for Marion to pick me up near Danie and Judy's home at a local petrol station. I pack up and move all my belongings to their home; when I return from Lily I have the opportunity to go on a safari with their organization and visiting Americans during the last week of my time in South Africa.

It is Sunday morning. A light drizzling rain falls as we wait for Marion to pick me up. A small silver Volkswagen Rabbit pulls alongside of Judy's car. Marion gets out and opens the hatchback while I unload my small luggage and backpack. Inside her car are bags of clothing, food, and paper products jammed into every corner. She moves some things and realizes even then there is no room for my luggage. She opens the passenger door and reveals the only space left, where I am to ride. I place my backpack on the floorboard, and climb in. Judy hands me my luggage and I place it on my lap. I recognize the concern on Judy's face as something I once would have felt, but I no longer judge circumstances. Instead, I look at everything as an adventure to be lived. And with a slam of the door, we are off.

We drive through Hilcrest and onto the N3 freeway, heading north I suppose. I had never traveled in this direction before. Typical housing developments and businesses of Hilcrest disappear. As the rolling hills known as the Valley of a Thousand Hills grow taller, the road steepens. The little car jammed to capacity with supplies weaves in and out of semi-trucks slowed by the terrain. On occasion, I can see further across the mountaintops than I had in months. Beautiful green rolling hills for as far as the eye could see.

I learn Marion is not the manager but is a registered nurse who volunteers at the children's village full time. Recovering from cancer, she has more work than she feels well enough to do. Lily of the Valley has 80 children living in small white cottages with green rooftops. Each cottage has a housemother and six children.

I smile when I realize I no longer think it odd we were driving on the left side of the road. My smile broadens when I realize there are many things I no longer take note of as my life continues to unfold before me. The car exits the freeway at the community of Hammersdale where most residents walk or take a twelve-passenger bus. Not only does our car stand out, so do the two white women riding in the front seat.

Marion travels to Lily three to five days per week, which contributes to her sense of confidence as we drive through Hammersdale past the stares of its residents. She chatters on about her work at Lily and those who call Lily home. The manager is a young man named Warren. He is single, but serves as father to eighty orphaned children.

The car slows and turns toward a road sign pointing to Mopelo. The road has a painted line down the center, but is too narrow for cars to pass without slowing to nearly a stop. We travel across the top of a grassy hilltop and drop down into a small community of simple block houses. There are no other cars, just an occasional bus. Today being Sunday, it seems most residents are strolling to church in what appears to be their Sunday finery. Young men wearing white crisp shirts and creased trousers, women wearing perfectly pressed dresses and hats, some carrying parasols. Children dart in and out of groups of people, often times out into the street.

As our car slows to the errant child or rebellious teen, the local residents stare as we pass. Often someone will wave and Marion waves back. We leave the township known as Mopelo and head up another hill where the road turns to gravel. We turn onto a dirt road and Marion points out the newly built community hall and vegetable tunnels.

We stop at a gate manned by a security guard with a white toothy smile. He opens the gate for us. Alongside the gate is a white security wall with the words Lily of the Valley Children's Village. A light drizzle is still falling. There is no one outside the white and green cottages. For a place where eighty children live, it is eerily quiet.

Marion drives up to the volunteer cottage and helps me bring my things inside. Rebecca, an English student spending a year between secondary school and college, is at the table with three children making painted handprints on white fabric for curtains. The cottage has two bedrooms, a bath, kitchen and living room. The windows are open and a cool breeze makes it feel chilly and damp for me. After months of hot, humid weather, South Africa is beginning to experience the early signs of fall. The warmest piece of clothing I brought is a sweater.

Marion takes me on a tour of the manager's office, medical clinic, preschool, and after school homework classroom. In the center of the twenty cottages, half yet to be filled, are play equipment, a salt-water pool and large unimproved sports field. Inside the medical clinic are cabinets with over-the-counter drugs and prescription drugs.

Marion begins to introduce me to the different drugs and what they are used for. She shows me the simple scratch pad listing treatment and date for each patient, along with the drug regimen for those infected with HIV. She explains that the housemothers know what the children need and when. There are children being treated for tuberculosis, infections and fevers. The clinic is open every day so house mothers can bring children who are sick. Marion was so happy I had come. I felt pride well up inside me. Here I am at an African orphanage, I thought to myself.

"I thought since you are a nurse, I would take some time off," Marion stated. "I've been sick myself, and thank God He's answered my prayer by sending you."

The prideful smile across my face remains unchanged, but inside I begin to recount what Marion had just said. I am going to take some time off; since you are a nurse you can fill in for me for a few days. Fill in for me for a few days . . . . fill in for me for a few days. I watch as her mouth continues to move, but I hear nothing more that she says. *What?* I silently ask. *You are asking me to direct the care of eighty children, many with diseases, multiple diseases that kill?*

Evidently my body language conveys a positive answer, because within minutes of unloading the contents of her Volkswagen Rabbit I watch her drive back out through the security gate and out of sight.

With a lump in my throat, I return to the volunteer cottage to unpack my few things, but am met by a housemother carrying a small child. A simple touch of my hand tells me she burns with fever. Carrying the clinic keys, we make our way back through the drizzling rain to the clinic where I begin what would be a long first day at Lily administering antibiotics, pain killers, anti-retro viral drugs to tiny children battling for their lives.

I realized early in the day, that whatever I feared was far less fearsome than anything these tiny children face: A deadly disease that already had a hold on their lives and wouldn't let go until it had won. On this first day, I discover these tiny children might have more courage than I.

During breaks in the steady stream of housemothers and children through the clinic doors, I notice children darting from cottage to cottage. When the sun breaks through, children fill the play structure accompanied by the universal and recognizable sound of recess.

Often times I look up from charting the treatment I gave the last visitor to see tiny faces with broad smiles of gleaming white teeth just barely tall enough to reach the window sill, peering in through the multiple panes of glass. With my wave, they scream and run away in laughter.

With the last of the late afternoon anti-retro viral cocktails administered, I close and lock the clinic and return to the volunteer cottage. Warren has offered to prepare a traditional Afrikaner (Af-re-cahn-er) meal called 'Toad in a Hole' casserole. (Afrikaners are Dutch descendants.) I am afraid to ask why it is called toad in a hole. The moment I cut into the baked muffin I discover the 'toad'. A chicken sausage baked in something similar to pancake batter. After weeks of chicken curried rice at the hospital, even a toad in a hole makes my taste buds celebrate.

Exhausted, I slump into an overstuffed chair and join Rebecca watching the equivalent to American daytime soap opera. Suddenly I realize there are many small frogs hopping across the floor. After weeks in South Africa I am accustomed to sharing my living space with cockroaches and ants, but not frogs.

"Oh, you don't have to worry about the frogs," Rebecca laughs. "It's the snakes coming in under the door after them you have to worry about! Don't sleep with your window open either. Not only will the mosquitos eat you alive, but the snakes can slither up the wall and in through your window!" I shudder.

After a hot bath in mineral stained water, I drift into a deep sleep. Early morning sunshine wakes me. With my eyes still closed I lay still and listen to the noises around me, attempting to determine where I am. Rolling over in bed reaching for my watch, I realize I have slept in. It is already 7:30. Somewhere I hear children's voices laughing and hollering as I swing my feet to the floor. I look down to see a small frog sitting atop one of my pink leather loafers stamped to look like crocodile. I think to myself, what a funny place this is. The thought of a frog sitting on a pink crocodile shoe in the middle of my room made me laugh.

Each morning Lily children gather around Warren's cottage in their navy sweater vests and slacks, and white blouses and plaid jumpers to make the five-mile trip to the local school. Warren makes several trips ferrying all school age children except those who are disabled or too sick to attend.

Within minutes of the children leaving, housemothers are hanging wash on outside lines, ferrying small toddlers to Lily's own preschool and enjoying conversation over an open back door. Often I hear them simply shout to one another from inside their cottage followed by a long "Yebo" (yes).

Most of the housemothers are Zulu mothers and gogos (grandmothers) to children of their own. They are often the only one employed in a large extended family, leaving their own families to raise the children of those who have died. Many of the housemothers have lost their adult children and husbands to AIDS, and are raising numerous grandchildren on their own. Being a housemother at Lily of the Valley is a highly prized job; many women will work as weekend replacements until a full-time position becomes available. Lily of the Valley housemothers are allowed one weekend off per month, and one month off per year.

In essence, these women become the mothers of children who have been orphaned or abandoned. They provide a home and family environment for the children, preparing meals, cleaning clothes and house. They attend to battles over toys, tears over scrapped knees, and everything that defines a normal childhood.

But life for these children has been far from normal even by South African standards. The loss of their mothers, fathers and siblings has decimated their lives. A young child is so closely associated with its mother that in the eyes of the child there is no distinction between the two. When a child loses its mother, the child loses its sense of identity.

When loss occurs at a young age, it can paralyze the developmental phases that build trust and autonomy in a young child.[8] If my mother who loved me leaves me, who else will leave me? This loss can produce fear instead of industry and independence in older children. The world is a scary place, where bad things happen to the people I love. The loss of something so dear as a child's mother may not only leave a cavernous hole in his heart, but also disable him emotionally.

One afternoon a housemother brings a small boy suffering with tuberculosis to the clinic. Marion had warned me that if the child's temperature exceeded 102 we needed to take him to a local clinic. He struggled to breathe between coughs and his temperature was over 103. We climb into the van, and one of Lily's drivers named Lucky drives us to a clinic about twenty minutes away. Lucky carries the small boy into an empty reception area where a woman is washing the floor. I stand at the open window of the empty office. I can hear voices but no one comes. Lucky holds the small boy as he shivers with fever.

The woman mopping the floor says the clinic is closed. "But we need to see a doctor," I replied. She props the mop handle against the wall and leaves. A woman wearing a nurse's uniform returns and I tell her, "I am a nurse volunteering at Lily of the Valley, and this small boy needs to see a doctor. He has tuberculosis and has a temperature of 103."

"I am sorry, but we are closed," she said in exhaustion.

"Marion told me you would see Lily children at the end of the day. I brought some chocolate Easter candy, if that will help," I persistently say. Marion's suggestion of bribery worked, and we are ushered into a treatment room.

During the second week, Marion returned. She decides it is a good time to conduct a health assessment on each of the children, especially the children who are HIV positive. Children qualified for anti-retro viral medication when a regular assessment documented a decline in the child's health over time. The assessments took days but would be worth the time if more children could qualify for drugs to treat the HIV and their diminished immunity.

Even though each day is exhausting, I attempt to make every moment count and visit the cottages in the evening when the children are bathed and ready for bed. I conduct toothbrush lessons with a coloring contest. Everyone wins with a new toothbrush donated by Oregon dentists, and their artwork hangs in the windows of the clinic.

One afternoon Warren asks if I will write thank you letters to all the children's sponsors. While going through the children's files I notice many had photographs tucked inside. Warren explained some of the photos are of sponsors, but some are actually the child's family members including mothers, fathers, and siblings.

As I write each letter on the computer I cannot stop thinking about how precious these keepsakes are, like a small window into a child's life. As I study the photographs, I grieve for the child whose life this photograph came from. I grieved for the mother looking back at me.

I thought of all the times I had cared for her child this week. The times I had held her child in my own arms, or watched as her child hollered to me from the top of the jungle gym, "Look at me, look at me!" Or laughed while colliding with others at the bottom of the slide, or soared into the sky feet first aboard a swing. Or cried with fever or ear infections. Or smiled through painful treatment of oozing carbuncles of the skin. Or the times spent simply sitting together in the sun on the back porch. I thought of this child who would never be held by their own mother again. And wept for his or her loss.

"Warren?" I ask. "What do you plan to do with the photos in the children's files?"

"I don't have any plans," he replies.

I explain to him that when each of Ron and my three sons graduated from high school, I created a scrapbook of childhood photographs and keepsakes stored in a box in the attic. While they looked through their books, they began to recount stories prompted by the photographs, awards, and schoolwork. Memories that would have likely been lost, had I not saved those priceless keepsakes over the years. Their scrapbooks play an important role in helping tell their own unique story and preserve their sense of identity.

"Warren, may I make the children their own scrapbooks to preserve their memories growing up at Lily?" I ask.

"Sure," he responds. I sense he doesn't understand, but he prints a list of all the children, and I set out to photograph each child so the child's name and photo could be on the first page of their scrapbook.

During several email exchanges with my sister Denyce back home, we discuss the possibility of women from her church in Lakeview, Oregon, assembling scrapbooks for all the children living at Lily. They would be simply decorated, but designed for the children to fill with keepsakes of their childhood. She agrees to oversee the purchase, design, and assembly of the scrapbooks. She suggests that the women at their summer retreat can put the scrapbooks together, and asks if I would consider coming to the retreat at Lake of the Woods to be the guest speaker. Of course I will! Denyce's enthusiasm for the project is infectious, and within days the committee planning the retreat agreed to the project to help the children in Africa. Neither they nor I would know then, these eighty scrapbooks would only be a beginning.

After an unbelievably busy and exhausting two weeks, the day I once longed for has arrived. But I did not want to leave what I have discovered here, what those who live here have taught me.

For the past two weeks, I have lived at the end of a dirt road far from home. I have had little in the way of clothing or food, and no communication with the outside world. Deadly sickness, dangerous animals, and loneliness have surrounded me. There have been moments when I felt so far from those I love and the life I live, yet in this place I am more myself than I have ever been before.

No façade or agenda to hide behind. No status or advantage. I am simply Ta-mar-ah, to the children of Africa. I have found the little one hidden inside of me, like the one who stares back at me from the deep brown eyes of the African child orphaned. Full of hope, dreams, healing like a bruised reed from life's cruelty and blindness to her needs.

I will truly never ever be the same. Lily of the Valley helped me write a chapter on the pages of my heart. No matter where we are, who we are, we are under the watchful gaze of a loving God who loves me enough to surprise me with the gift of not only discovering myself, but also finding I am deeply loved by God simply because I'm me.

I have discovered the answer to why all this suffering in this devastatingly beautiful place. I had to come to Africa to discover that suffering is the only way I would ever need or seek God.

I silently cry as Marion and I drive away from Lily on the dirt road that brought me here. I taste against my lips the salt left behind from hundreds of goodbye kisses and realize it is a perfect metaphor for life.

Chapter 8

More Than Just Words

It is Friday evening, and I have returned to Mercykton from my two weeks at Lily. Danie and I are sitting at the kitchen counter snacking on cashews while I convey the terror when a Lily housemother finds a Black Mamba under a baby crib. Judy has just returned from decorating for the weekend school dance, and heads upstairs to change for dinner when she discovers someone in the house attempting to steal their valuables. Judy screams, 'push the panic button, Danie! Someone's in the house!'

The authorities fail to find the person before fleeing through an upstairs window. Danie arranges for 24-hour security, but I fear the security person may not be trusted. And apparently neither do Danie and Judy as they suggest I sleep in the guest room next to theirs.

After the frightful night, I sit under a large umbrella next to the pool, comforted by a cup of hot rooibos tea. A snoozing security guard is sitting nearby in the shade of a large tree. The irony of the break-in is that for weeks I have stayed at McCord Hospital locked behind the door of the doctor's quarters because of the threat of crime. I just spent weeks at Lily of the Valley on the outskirts of a township where white South African people never ever would travel to or through because of the threat of crime.

Yet, here in this place I have come for sanctuary, the threat of crime becomes real. I wonder how people live with this kind of danger everyday. I wonder what the physical, emotional toll must be. How do people face these kinds of threats everyday without succumbing to a constant state of fear? What are the long-term effects on the children who witness the violence?

As I reflect on this event, I realize it is the story of apartheid in South Africa except the roles of white and black are reversed. Black South Africans lived with danger every day, with great physical and emotional toll and faced threats everyday simply because of their skin color. Discrimination, violence, and bondage have inflicted devastating long-term effects on generations of South Africans, including its children. I find myself humming a song I recently learned here in South Africa, simply allowing the words to cross my mind.

> God bless Africa, God bless Africa.
> Guide her leaders, guard her children,
> And give her peace.
>
> Nkosi sikelel iAfrica, Nkosi sikelel iAfrica,
> Guide her leaders, guard her children,
> And give her peace.[9]

Will there ever be a day this refrain will be more than just words? Will there ever be a time all South Africans live together in peace? Maybe it will begin with the children.

Chapter 9

Filling an Empty Space

One last time I turn to wave goodbye to my friends Danie and Judy and continue to walk across the tarmac to my awaiting flight home. Something was strangely different from the last time I boarded a plane when all I felt was a dreadful ache in my chest. When I arrived months ago, the pain I felt was for myself. Today, the heartache is for others. Those I have come to admire love and cherish, the South Africans who now hold a place in my heart, who I will never, ever forget. As I watch the orange soil of Africa disappear from beneath the plane, I believe somehow I will return. There is a saying in Africa: once the dust of Africa covers the soles of your shoes, you will never forget her whereever you go. I spend the time flying home reading and rereading my journal, adding additional comments and final assessments of my time in Africa.

I read about the day I was driven to a local informal hospice operated by four nurses. I thought of the young woman who was dying of AIDS while her small child played near her feet covered with a white crisp sheet. I thought about the housemother at Lily, Big Martha, who came to the volunteer cottage one afternoon. She said she once heard me say God sees her. He knows all her good deeds. That she is never alone because God is always near. She wanted to know if that was true. I assured her it was. She sobbed in my arms.

I was reminded about the frightful night I was asked to drive in South Africa for the first time on the left hand side of the street, with twelve children and several volunteers in a large van. Our destination was Pietermaritzburg to attend an Anglican Church service. I'll never forget when we filed into the church already filled with white South Africans, and filled one entire pew with smiling black faces. When the communion plate was passed all eyes watched as the happy children took a cup and small wafer without knowledge of religious doctrine or their violation therein, but were simply happy for the 'refreshments' served. I smiled knowing Jesus implored the adults to 'let the children come' and left feeling no guilt whatsoever.

I was so grateful to return to the Phinda Game Reserve where Ron and I had enjoyed a traditional safari the year before. I loved sleeping in the Forest Camp where cottage walls were made entirely of glass, and the black obsidian rock shower was outside. I loved waking to small Vervet monkeys sitting in a nearby tree, and tiny red Dika antelope grazing under brush. Game rangers escort you to and from your cottage because wild animals roamed freely as this was their home.

I enjoyed the hot rooibos tea and biscuit picnic while we waited for the elephants to come to water as dawn broke. I loved the game drives searching for cheetah, rhinoceros, hippos, various antelope like the springbok, and the funny warthogs. Walter, my game ranger, told me that the phrase, "Let's high tail it out of here," came from warthogs. I laughed every time I saw a shy warthog run from view with its tail straight in the air. Or the origin of the dung beetle name because it rolled balls of dung many times its weight into a waiting hole where it laid its eggs. Walter asked if I noticed the absence of dung across the African plain. He was right. There was none.

At night female lions successfully took down a magnificent giraffe while the pride's male watched. Dominant males preserve their strength and endurance so they can defend and maintain their pride from younger male lions.

The black African sky was filled with millions upon millions of stars, and Walter pointed to the Southern Cross used by explorers for centuries to locate due south. I loved the night we drove into the bush and came upon brown paper lanterns lighting the way to a beautiful dinner with fine china, silver, wine glasses, and a gourmet meal. Zulu warriors danced around a raging bonfire. The dust rising created an eerie illusion as they spun and stomped in the tradition of their forefathers.

I remembered the night a full moon rose overhead, and the thought came to me, Ron will see the same moon tomorrow night. When we spoke I told him to watch for Mr. Moon; he is bringing a message of my love.

Etched in my mind is the day I roamed about Sinikithemba at day's end, hoping to see those I had worked along side of, grown to love through friendship to say my good-byes. It felt fitting there was no one there. The reception room was quiet with only echoes of voices from somewhere inside the offices behind. The examination rooms, the lab, the training and staff meeting rooms were empty except for two students on a computer. It felt fitting this wasn't good-bye, for I knew deep within it wasn't. As I turned to leave, I saw the young man I met on my first day in South Africa at the Dream Center sitting in a wheelchair at the curb. Next to him an elderly woman sat on the pavement of the sidewalk. As I walked toward him, I realized he had seen me long before I recognized him. A smile broke out across his face immediately. "Oh my goodness!" I smiled. "I am so happy to see you." I reached out my hand toward his extended hand. Like most Zulu speaking South Africans, he understood English more than he could speak it. His body language spoke volumes. "How are you doing?" I asked. He shook his head, yet still smiled. I extended my right hand to the woman he introduced as his mother, placing my left hand on top my right arm just below the elbow, signifying I come in peace in Zulu. She humbly lowered her head, but gripped my hand firmly.

What do you say to a man whom you may never see again? Whom you know is battling for his life? While once awkward, the silence between us filled with something more important than words—a sense of shared understanding about the human condition. My body may be dying around me, but I am a person inside. While the odor of this death may be overpowering, will you share these last days of my life with me? Will you stop and say hello?

"May I pray for you?" I asked him. Yes. Yes, please he shakes his head. As I kneel on the pavement with their hands in mine, I offer a prayer to God for this man and his mother in this place called hope. When I open my eyes, I see tears streaming down his face and realize this moment was from God for both of us; the space between living and dying where only loving matters.

After a long journey home, I fall into the arms of a loving family beginning with the most eager, my two grandchildren. With tear stained face, my mother Jean waits her turn. I attempt to fight back tears as each of my sons and beautiful daughters-in-law come forward; Joshua lifts the heavy backpack from my travel weary shoulders. And finally Ron, his embrace never wanting to leave. While many friends and family have spoken of my sacrifice to go to Africa, the truth is that Ron paid a greater sacrifice by letting me go. And I love him even more for his selflessness.

Following days of fighting off jetlag, I begin to slowly reenter the life I left that continued as usual while I was away. I immediately take over the care giving of my mother and enjoy time with my family and friends. Yet, inside I am confronted by a great battle. Would I deny the changes I experienced while in Africa and simply slip back into the person I once was? No one could know from the outside I had changed. The things important to me had changed. I began to wonder if I would ever fit back into the space I once lived.

Last year, Dr. Holst suggested I come to Africa and volunteer. Not only did it not ease from my mind what I saw there, but now after volunteering for three months I feel more compelled by what I cannot forget—thousands upon thousands of children losing everything dear to them. Never being held by their mothers again.

I ask myself: *Would I ever be the same?* Inside a quiet voice replies, *I hope not.*

Chapter 10

A Place to Tell Their Stories

During the summer retreat, I join Lakeview Baptist Church women to assemble the personalized scrapbooks for the eighty children living at Lily. While sitting in small groups, women and young girls apply letter stickers spelling out the child's name across the front of the individual scrapbook they are creating. Tears well up in the eyes of women as they study the photo of the child to whom the book belongs. A handmade monogrammed white handkerchief is neatly folded and placed on the last page. Quietly, women pen a letter of love and encouragement to the child and place it in the back of the book. When all books are complete, a group photo is taken with the women holding the book each created. The photo will be placed in the book prior to shipping them to South Africa.

In the midst of assembling these scrapbooks, those who so lovingly touch and assemble each aspect of the scrapbook are moved by the message this gift will be to a child. The messages on the scrapbook pages tell that God knew them before they were born. God made them wonderfully. God has a plan and purpose for their life. God even knows their name!

Inspired to conclude the retreat with a gift for each woman, I invite each one to stand one by one and read the meaning of their names. With tears often streaming down their faces, I realize God is healing the wounded child-like hearts of the women at the same time He has invited us to join Him in helping heal the wounds of orphaned children in Africa.

While excited to know the children at Lily will enjoy and benefit from having a scrapbook to store their childhood keepsakes, I openly wonder while running with friend Stacy whether other children would benefit by having a scrapbook. During quiet moments of gardening throughout the summer, my thoughts are filled with memories of South Africa and thoughts for the possibility of shipping more scrapbooks to children.

I am unable to quiet those thoughts, and wonder if it is an invitation from God to not only never forget the African children, but also to see the path that led me to Africa last year continue on and out of sight. I wait for the familiar quiet voice to come. The voice I learned to recognize as not my own. Quietly I wait, but there is only silence.

South Africa

After months in the hold of an ocean-going freighter and journey by train, truck, and eventually ferrying by Noel and Pat Wright, board members for Lily, eighty Memory Books arrive for the children who call Lily of the Valley their home. I can only imagine the excitement when the children realize the gift they hold in their hands has been uniquely made just for them. On the front cover reads their name spelled out in stickers, and on the front page under their name and birthdate is their individual photograph with a place to tell their story.

The children's village volunteers organize the first of many opportunities for the children to make a keepsake for their Memory Book. With paper plates filled with orange, blue, red, and green paint the children place their hands in the paint and then onto a page inside their Memory Book devoted to handprints. The page describes our handprints as unique to each one of us, none being the same.

I receive word from Pat as to the joyous arrival of the Memory Books, but am deeply saddened to learn that two of the children at Lily have died during the past few months. Pat wanted to know what to do with their unused Memory Books. In honor of their lives, I suggest the memory books be tied with a white ribbon and placed somewhere as a memorial to the significance of their lives. Volunteers paint a mural of a garden on the wall of the clinic where the Memory Books are placed. Butterflies, flowers, bumble bees, and other garden inhabitants are given the names of each child who has died at Lily. It becomes a public and constant reminder of the value of every child who has called Lily home.

While news of the Memory Books arrival and welcome reception is extremely satisfying, I am overwhelmed with the news of the children who have died and grieve deeply for each of them. I am convinced no one is braver than a child who courageously lives apart from his mother. I think of the day a child realizes they no longer must endure separation, and may even welcome the rest of death. I do not know. I can only imagine the moment a child is swept into the loving arms of his mother, finally home for all eternity, as one of the greatest of joys.

Chapter 11

Un-regrettable Epitaph

I would return to Africa by any invitation. When we received an invitation to climb Mt. Kilimanjaro, Ron enthusiastically agreed. We will join a friend, Rochelle Sittko, and a group from Denver, Colorado, climbing for charity. She knew of our lifelong dream to summit the tallest mountain on the continent after friends reported it "a walk-up" and we felt the opportunity might never come again.

After months of training on the stair machine and acquiring the necessary equipment needed for high altitude climbing, Ron and I boarded the long flight through Frankfurt, Germany, and onto Nairobi in Kenya. From there we board a small plane that is going to take us across the border into Tanzania where Kilimanjaro straddles the border between the two countries. Economically dwarfed by Kenya, the border between the countries was moved to give Tanzanian's opportunity to prosper by a climbing and tourist industry.

From the right side of the plane, I see an enormous mountain ahead and surmise it to be Kilimanjaro. Inside my stomach begins to churn when I face the fear I had ignored earlier. *Am I really capable of climbing Mt. Kilimanjaro?*

The pilot's voice interrupts my thoughts and points out Kilimanjaro. But to my amazement he suggests we look out the left side of the plane. From my seat, I can only see the lower half of the mountain we would be climbing. The small mountain to our right dwarfed in comparison to towering Kilimanjaro that jets 19,340 feet from the African desert floor, the highest freestanding mountain in the world.

I elbow Ron. "Look at that mountain!" I shudder.

We land at Kilimanjaro International Airport, a one-room terminal to facilitate the daily plane with twenty-four passengers from Nairobi. Inside we meet Wilderness Travel Head Guide Godson (Sekay) and an assistant guide, John. We recognize others from the plane. Team members from Denver include Steve, John with son Derrick, 15, and Kathleen, 16, daughter of the charity's founder. Our friend Rochelle is flying in tomorrow.

We will spend two days resting and acclimating at a campsite outside the town of Arusha at the foot of Mt. Meru (14,000 ft). The mountain I mistakenly thought was Kili. We enjoy gourmet meals prepared by chefs who will accompany us on the climb. Porters pour a bucket of hot water into the portable shower attached to our tent and we enjoy the first shower in days. We take short walks, and a game drive at dusk.

Sekay has summited Kilimanjaro one hundred times. He comes to each of our individual tents and inventories all of the necessary equipment we were to bring to secure his 100% rate of success for all clients. He quizzes us about our plan to utilize medication, Diamox, for high altitude sickness. Living at nearly sea level, Ron and I make the decision to take Diamox that will increase the amount of oxygen the blood can store.

Sekay stresses the importance of following directions of the guides, and being completely honest to him about how we are doing physically and mentally. Hiding symptoms is deadly at high elevations. I quietly worry that the cold symptoms I brought won't subside once we enter the cold and altitude of the mountain.

Rochelle arrives in camp after dark and reports armed men confronted the driver and her as they entered the park.

It's New Year's Eve the night before we begin our climb. What a way to start a new year! Sitting around a bonfire, we tell stories about our lives, and our climbing experiences to one another and then retire earlier than on most New Year's celebrations. Neither Ron nor I sleep well. We wake exhausted the day of the six-hour drive to the foot of Mt. Kilimanjaro. Ron suffers from a runny tummy (a term some Africans use for diarrhea) and begins taking medication he would eventually need for the entire climb. The sore throat I came with has developed into body aches and a headache. It's like the marathons I have run; all the training in the world cannot prevent waking on race day to illness that changes everything.

The caravan of land cruisers begins the journey across flat grassless land dotted with dwarf thorny acacia trees. The dirt road before us crosses dry ditches and slows for cow and goatherds driven by long stick-toting boys. With a short grass broom, a woman stoops to sweep debris across the dirt surrounding a small brick house while children interrupt their game of chasing one another to watch our convoy pass. It is hot and dusty with water nowhere to be found.

Kilimanjaro remains in front of us until we begin the slow ascent up the hills that flank its enormous circumference. We pass fields planted with coffee bushes, cypress trees, tall grass fields, and small communities of homes. Everyone walking, even children, appear to be carrying water. Two small boys push a small wooden block with wheels with a long attached stick; other children chase beside them laughing. Girls dressed in pink and white dresses stare as we drive by, responding with shy grins when they see me waving.

After Sekay registers us to climb Kilimanjaro at the gate of the park, the jeeps begin a steep ascent up deeply rutted muddy roads where we meet up with the rest of our climbing team; fifty-seven guides, porters, and cooks for the seven of us. I laugh when I realize we each would have a personal porter to carry our duffel bag of personal equipment. I would only be required to carry a daypack with items I might need during the day.

As we leave the parked vehicles and begin a steep climb through dense forested vegetation, I immediately begin to sweat and am short of breath. I secretly wonder if I am already in over my head. Every few minutes a porter carrying a huge bundle atop his head passes us calling out "pollie, pollie" (slow and steady). I begin to respond to each of them in Swahili "asanti-san" (thank you very much).

The first day ends after six miles and we are still amidst the forested hillsides. We come upon a small city of tents set up by several other climbing groups. Our porters immediately lift our daypacks from our shoulders and hand us a hot cup of tea, a tradition we will soon relish as temperatures begin to lower the higher we climb.

Porters lead us across Forest Camp and direct us to our own tent where our duffel bags lay, both a man's and woman's portable tented toilet and the crown jewel of this moving city, the mess tent. During the next few days, we learn that a fully outfitted mess tent with tables, chairs, lanterns, and delicious hot meals is not the norm. Wilderness Travel excursions are the envy of everyone we meet. I actually feel a bit guilty when we discover two Australian climbers who had just arrived from Australia that day and were suffering jetlag, high altitude, and cold cheese sandwiches all at once.

After tomato ginger soup and chicken with peanut sauce over coconut rice for dinner, the last thing I remember before drifting off to sleep is Steve hollering at us to open our tent door to what else, but twinkling Christmas lights strung across his tent. Surely a New Year's Day to remember!

Up early and back on the trail, the climb takes us away from the tall trees and thick undergrowth and we begin to follow a ridgeline saddle that slowly rises to an unobstructed view of a cloud-shrouded Kilimanjaro. With my eyes glued to the vista overhead I don't see the surprise before me until I nearly fall over a perfectly decorated table set for lunch, complete with linens, folding chairs, and a beautiful meal. Once again I laugh at the novelty of it all.

As we dine during a lunch break, porters, often wearing simple canvas shoes, continue to run past, carrying an amazing amount of equipment atop their heads. We all howl in laughter when Sekay calls out to the egg man—a young man carrying a wire basket filled with 400 eggs atop his head and running carefully. He smiles knowing his job is especially important. For the next ten days we would learn that each of the fifty-seven men and young boys have a role to play in ferrying fifty pounds of gear to the top of this African continent, the summit of Kilimanjaro.

That evening we arrive at Shira Camp at 11,000 ft. where our personal tents are set up. Dinner is already being prepared outside the mess tent. After washing up with warm water, we don parkas, hats, and glove liners for the first time. The unabated icy wind chills me. Sekay demonstrates the use of a high altitude sickness chamber designed to increase blood oxygen levels of someone suffering the debilitating and deadly affliction of high altitude sickness. Sekay questions each of us throughout the day and at meals in an attempt to diagnose symptoms of high altitude sickness.

The Australians have arrived in camp and one of the climbers is suffering from severe headache, the first indication of high altitude sickness. Their travel group has limited accommodations and meager rations. We offer him painkillers and suggest he increase his water intake.

The wind continues and blows all night. There is no warmth but one's own body heat. Proper clothing and gear is vital at this elevation, and considered life saving the higher we climb. Without the warmth that hiking produces, I wear most of my gear while in camp, including gloves during meals.

The next day the hike is shortened, giving us a chance to acclimate at Scott Fischer Camp, named after the famed owner of Mountain Madness climbing company in Seattle who died on Mt. Everest in 1996. Scott loved climbing Kilimanjaro and donated hundreds of hiking boots to porters and guides. Sekay shows us a plaque honoring Scott.

We arrive early in the day, which allows us time to relax. A damp fog has rolled in and reduces visibility to nothing. I climb into our tent with a cup of hot cocoa and my journal. In the quietness of our tent, I read through a small devotional book and am reminded of God's presence even in this remote place of His creation.

I write in my journal the words I hear. *In the greatness of this place, the mightiness and magnificence of this mountain, my love for you is even greater. Can you imagine? As great as this place is, greater is my love for you. When you step upon this great mountain I want you to remember the beautiful and delicate alpine flower tucked away in the crevice of the rock is my creation and placed here by me. It has fulfilled its purpose, high atop this sometimes-inhospitable mountain, when you see that you, too, can survive life's storms.*

The next morning we leave Fischer Camp for the easy hike to the 15,000-foot camp at Lava Tower. Leaving the heather mountain zone behind, we enter a barren landscape where nothing but small grasses sprout, and lichen and mosses cling to volcanic rock. The sky is cobalt blue.

Just before we arrive at Lava Tower, porters run past us up hill carrying a rolled canvas stretcher. They speak to Sekay in Swahili without stopping. I surmise someone is sick and must be carried off the mountain. When high altitude sickness affects a climber, an immediate retreat to lower altitude is critical to reverse the deadly symptoms.

We arrive at Lava Tower at noon amidst warmth of full sunshine and pull mess tent chairs outside into the sun, oblivious to the absence of activity at camp. Dozens of our porters can be seen running up the trail toward tomorrow's camp at 17,500 feet. It is well past lunchtime, yet nothing is being prepared. I begin to miss the normal attentiveness of my porter and question where he is.

Clouds move in and darken the sky. The warmth of this beautiful day is about to change. Sekay joins us and says it is a sad day on the mountain; after a large rockslide three Americans and many porters are dead. Many, many are injured.

Anxiety grows within and overwhelms me as the injured begin to enter our camp. Some are bleeding from head and leg wounds. Others have suffered broken legs, shoulders, and arms. Dining chairs and sleeping bags are dragged in front of the mess tent where Sekay begins to treat the wounded with bandages until supplies are gone. Splints are made from hiking poles and strips of torn clothing while we attempt to comfort the climbers who have witnessed this tragedy.

A badly hurt couple from Denver limps into camp. Through a quaking voice she reports, "There was the sound of rocks falling, then we saw a rockslide coming down above us. The slide began to pick up speed and size. There was no place to hide. We were in the direct path of falling rocks the size of cars. There were 150 climbers, guides and porters on the trail. A woman took a direct hit by a passing boulder and lay motionless down the hillside. I knew she was dead. No one could survive anything like that."

Two college age children arrive. We stand stunned and in shock as porters carry a canvas stretcher into camp carrying the body of their mother, her grief stricken husband following close behind the procession. Her body is covered with a green wool blanket, but her brown leather boots left visible. I quietly gasp when I look down to realize she and I wore the same boots. I shudder in disbelief and panic, realizing that could have been me. That could be me lying dead on a stretcher. I silently wonder: *What am I doing on the side of this mountain?*

Porters continue to carry sleeping bags into our camp; inside those who had died. Another stretcher carried a porter suffering a compound fracture of the femur and in shock. Our porters run up and down the trail to 17,500 feet where the accident happened well after dark, making sure everyone makes it down. Their own grief over the tragedy of lost friends is quietly shared among one another. Unfortunately, it would be another three-mile hike down to Shira Camp where rescue vehicles will transport the injured to a hospital in Moshi. I cannot imagine the agony of following the stretcher carrying their mother. This is supposed to be a "walk up."

After Steve calls home using his satellite phone, we take turns calling our families. We realize the news of the rockslide with fatalities of Americans will shock our children. And it did! They had already heard about the accident and were making plans for our eldest son, Jeff, to fly to Nairobi. They were relieved to hear from us, but were admittedly terrified. I grieved knowing they suffered thinking we might be dead.

Sekay calls us to the mess tent for a team meeting. All reports from Wilderness Travel offices tell him the trail above us is impassable and too dangerous to use. The first reports are that the warm temperatures melted the glacier cornice near the summit, resulting in the rockslide. Three Americans from New York and Denver were killed, with an unknown number of porters losing their lives. Our options are to either abandon our climb or circumvent the mountain and summit using the more popular direct route. The two additional days of hiking would require us to climb from 15,000 feet to the summit at 19,340 feet and then retreat to 10,000 feet in one day. My immediate reaction is to get off this mountain! But we agree to think about it over night. Frankly, I had lost the motivation necessary to continue. Life is precious, but climbing this mountain isn't, I said. Sekay said no one would need to continue against their wishes; there is enough staff that anyone can be escorted down the mountain.

Thinking of the woman's boots, I sensed God asking me: *Are you ready for the last day of your life? Are you living each day as though it is your last?* What a profound and sobering question for us all.

With no appetite for food, I climb into the comfort of our tent alone and am sickened to think of the tragedy we witnessed. A wave of sorrow overcomes me. I fumble through my pack for my small devotional Bible and begin to read through tear-blurred vision from the page to which it opens. *At your side one thousand people may die, or even ten thousand, right beside you, but you will not be hurt. The Lord is your protection; you have made God Most High your place of safety. Nothing bad will happen to you; no disaster will come to your home.* (Psalm 91:7-10, my paraphrase)

I am reminded of my earlier encounter when seeing the tiny alpine flower tucked away in the crevice of a rock. I feel comforted and thankful knowing that God can also protect me, just as He protects the flower.

Beneath ink black skies and millions upon millions of stars, we exit our tent at 11 p.m. in the midst of stiff winds and sub-freezing temperatures. For two days we circumvent the mountain, gaining and losing elevation. We arrive at Barafu Camp (meaning icy cold) where we find our tents assembled among many, many other teams. Extreme cold and constant icy wind replaces distance and elevation gain as the nemesis to our goal.

Led by Sekay, John, and our personal porters, we begin the final climb to the summit of Kilimanjaro. The team has been noticeably quiet over the past two days of hiking, with an absence of laughter and practical jokes that previously accompanied us. Witnessing the loss of life of fellow Americans and the young porters and guides defines the priority of summiting this pile of rock for each of us. I couldn't care less, but recognize I may never be in this place again. Maybe over time accomplishing the goal Ron and I had dreamt of would ease the pain of tragedy. Once again I hear, *Am I living life each day as if it were my last?*

The warm yellow lights of headlamps from hundreds of climbers dance like fireflies in a steady stream above us. Without even a sliver of moon overhead, my headlamp is all that illumines each rock where my porter has just stepped, and I move upward. Ron steps where my boot once set and his porter follows close behind. The wind howls; within minutes I stop to put on additional clothing and insulated gloves over the glove liners. Ron does the same and realizes one of the fingers of his glove is sewn shut. After failing to get the glove on, his porter takes off his gloves and gives them to Ron. His porter pushes his hands into his blue jeans and waves for us to continue.

One step up after another, through the darkness, through the cold and wind, there is no way of measuring how far we have come or have to go. So we simply continue to take one step after another. Our warm breath form frozen mustaches beneath our noses and icicles across the zippered opening of our jackets. Any attempt to stop and rest is quickly abandoned when the heat from our activity evaporates immediately. The melodious rhythm of my breathing distracts me from the monotony of stepping up, and I hum a rhythmic melody inside my head.

With my head down focusing on the next step, I fail to see the sky beginning to lighten and Kilimanjaro now silhouetted overhead. To my amazement, I discover we have been climbing for seven hours. We stop when the sun breaks the horizon and climbs quickly above the African plain. I smile when I realize we couldn't possibly be far from the summit; I take another step up.

Ahead I see many climbers congregated and wonder if there is something wrong. My porter turns to me and reports, "We're here! You've made it to the summit of Kilimanjaro!" What? I thought. I am confused. This is the summit? I looked around I realized no one was stepping up rocks anymore. The ground beneath me was simply sand. I turned to Ron and cried. Stuttering, I said, "We've made it. We've finally made it to the summit of Kilimanjaro," as I bury my head against his shoulder.

In wilderness travel style, after climbing to 19,340 feet, my porter, with a smile, pulls from his backpack a thermos and hands each of us a cup of hot tea. We watched as other members of our team arrive with the same reaction, "This is the summit?" They question. "Yes, this is the summit!"

Enormous glaciers standing five stories tall and etched by deep blue ice crevasses skirt the summit. It has been many years since Kilimanjaro has been covered with snow. We hike an additional quarter mile across the sand to the true summit before we descend to escape the unbearable cold.

It took eight days of climbing to reach the summit and eight hours to glissade down 10,000 feet through sifting rock and sand. Arriving at Barafu Camp, we find hot tomato soup and grilled cheese sandwiches made especially for us after our porters reported what we dreamt of while climbing to the summit.

Ron and I spend a day recovering at a beautiful retreat once a coffee plantation in Arusha. I stand in a hot shower until fatigue wins out. We sip Orange Crush from glass bottles and nap under the mosquito netting atop a crisp white duvet. The simple things of life are made special by their absence.

In the days following, we caravan across the Serengeti and the Ngorongoro Crater and complete our trip to Tanzania. The words I heard on the day of Kilimanjaro's worst climbing disaster in history keep invading my thoughts. *Are you ready for the last day of your life? Am I? Have I lived every moment as though it might be my last? I think about the battle I faced when I returned home after volunteering in Africa. Would I simply slip back into a life focused on myself? If that would be my choice, would I regret the day my life ends? Or what if I choose to live my life for others? What regret would there be in that?*

Chapter 12

A Story of Instinct

Ron and I are home from Tanzania for less than a month before I board a flight to South Africa with Katie, a college student from the church youth group with which Ron and I were involved. Inside a darkened plane of sleeping travelers, I pace the aisles for hours, holding back tears. After the climbing disaster, all I want is to be home, safe and secure with those I love. Yet I am returning to Lily of the Valley to fulfill a promise to Katie and to God. I truly want to know what has happened to the scrapbooks. But I just wish there was some other way.

In the days leading up to our departure, I pray and ask God to show me how I can know if I am being led by Him or if I am simply obsessed by my own desire to go back to Africa. I decide I would begin to read the Bible until I heard His answer. Within a few days, I read Exodus 2 and the story about a child born during the time when all Jewish newborn boys were to be killed to satisfy a ruler's insecurity about his power. The mother abandons the child in a basket along the bank of the river, knowing this action may be the child's only hope of survival.

I realize as I read and reread the story of Moses that every woman is moved to care for him, even at her own peril. From the midwives instructed to drown newborn Jewish baby boys to Moses' mother Jochebed and even his older sister Miriam, each woman risked her own life to save the life of the child.

Was this the answer I was looking for? That God endows every female with a maternal instinct to protect and preserve the life of a child? Truly, that instinct is evident in all creation. God created a way for the most vulnerable among us to be rescued in time of need, and it lies within each one of us. I cried when I realized this was God's answer to my question. He has already created a way to help vulnerable children. If only the cries of African children could be heard a world away.

Africa. Her green rolling hills are familiar enough to feel like home. The Valley of a Thousand Hills is the same today as yesterday. Nothing has changed except my perspective. As we drive down the dirt road toward Lily's gate I feel as though I am coming home to my African life. Judy and Danie have retrieved us from the airport, helped us gather a few groceries and driven us north through Mopelo. Lily is our base from which we will make plans to go wherever opportunity leads us. Depending on how the scrapbooks have been received by Lily children, I am driven by the thought there certainly must be other children who would enjoy having a personal scrapbook of their own.

Immediately our volunteer cottage is filled with children curious about our arrival. But I realize many of those children I recognize do not remember me. Many volunteers have come and gone during the last year. And life has gone on while I have been away. A small girl once had long black hair that distinguished her from others with their short-cropped hair. Today she, too, has short hair. Another child who had been extremely ill last year appears to have weathered that storm, and several young boys have grown so much I do not immediately recognize them. While playing, a small girl I recognize looks deeply into my eyes and begins to smile when she realizes I am Ta-mar-ah!

Waking after only a couple hours of sleep, I lay in the darkness until I hear the birds announcing a new day. Traveling through ten time zones takes ten days to fully adjust. As I lay in bed I think about the prospects for scrapbooks and whether I could actually find 1,000 children in need of one. *Oh my, how will it happen? Surely, if this truly is God's idea He certainly knows.*

For days we join the daily activities of Lily, and Katie joins the ranks of a dozen students from England doing whatever is needed—mostly mundane chores, such as those that define life anywhere in the world. One by one, housemothers erupt in shouts of glee when they realize I have returned and greet me with open arms. On our first Sunday, the salt-water pool is opened and immediately fills with children donning bright orange "water wings." Katie and I join in the melee.

That evening we walk up the dirt road to the volunteer house near the community center to have dinner with a U.S. couple and their three young and beautiful blonde daughters. They belong to a church that sponsors children living at Lily. The husband produces music and has brought equipment to Lily to produce CD's of the Lily children singing. Dressed in a lovely white, layered skirt, African print tank, long necklaces and bracelets, with trundles of her blonde hair escaping from a bun, the wife describes their first month in South Africa. The girls come and go from the table. The wife continues to tell us how they had decided to leave their life in Southern California and live in South Africa for two years. As words flowed from her mouth, I hear nothing because my mind is racing with thoughts of danger. Danger ahead I silently shout! Danger! Danger! I wonder if they are blinded by the romance of coming to Africa and are completely unaware of how dangerous this place may be for all of them, especially their beautiful daughters. Last year, I was horrified to learn of the myth many African men believe: they will be cured of HIV/AIDS by having intercourse with a virgin.

Suddenly she turns to me, "Tell me about you."

"What?" I realize she is addressing me. "I am married and have three sons," I respond almost automatically from the fog of my daydream. Inside, my thoughts are screaming: *Do you know how dangerous it is here? Do you know how dangerous it is to have your beautiful daughters here? This home doesn't even have a fence or wall. What will happen when people find out you have this expensive electronic equipment? How will you protect your children? Yourselves?*

The uncomfortable silence is broken by a knock on the door. A security guard from Lily tells the husband to come, as he has discovered Warren's cottage has been ransacked while he is away for a few days. Through the darkness, the security guard shines a flashlight on a large hole cut in the ten-foot tall cyclone fencing directly behind Warren's cottage back door. Inside we discover an empty space where television, microwave, and other appliances once were.

Woof! Woof! Woof! The distant sound of bloodhounds fill the darkness. Woof! Woof! Rumbling into the Lily yard, an old farm pickup truck filled with barking dogs and men standing in the truck bed. A white man wearing a white sleeveless t-shirt, overalls, and toting a rifle climbs from behind the wheel and places the barrel of his gun directly on the toe of his steel-toed boot. With a strong Africaans (Dutch dialect) accent, he shouts questions over the noise of the barking dogs.

Woof! Woof! The bloodhounds bellow.

"How long ago did the break in happen?" he shouts. The security guard explains Warren has been gone for days. Woof! Woof! It could have been hours or days. The man shouts in Zulu to the black men holding the dogs. They immediately jump from the bed of the truck and unleash the dogs. Woof! Woof! Instinctively, the dogs take off through the hole in the fence, their noses to the ground, and disappear into the darkness, followed by the men.

"The dogs 'el get 'em if they're still roun'," he smirks through a large gap between his front teeth. The Afrikaner farmer came from a long line of Dutch immigrants of both rebellious and self-reliant citizenry— determined to take care of their own problems out here.

Chapter 13

Defining South Africa's Future

Stacked on shelves, divided by age, I find the children's scrapbooks in Warren's office. Taking one to a nearby chair, I open it to find the child's photograph on the front page followed by pages filled with beautiful childhood keepsakes; small painted handprints, drawings, photographs, and school awards fill the pages. After only one year, a child's life story is already being preserved and told, intricate memories otherwise undoubtedly lost over time. Volunteers, staff, and the children themselves have all contributed to the contents of their books.

Two young boys join me, anxiously remove their own scrapbooks from the shelf, and eagerly show me the contents. As they turn each page, I watch the expression across their faces as they describe drawings and read stories. They laugh at one another's photographs; at times they appear to become reflective as they quietly reread salutations across the bottoms of greeting cards.

The office fills with children wanting to show me their scrapbooks. I agree to visit each of their cottages in the evening and bring their scrapbooks so we can look at them one at a time. For the next several evenings, when everyone is fed, bathed, and ready for bed, I bring scrapbooks for each child in a cottage and sit close looking at the contents with each and every child. All around the room children's faces are buried in the pages of their personal scrapbooks and the memories that define their lives. The housemother is unaware of the children's scrapbooks stored in the office for safekeeping, and covers her tear-stained face with her apron.

Before I leave I ask the children to draw pictures of themselves using paper and crayons I brought. For some of the tiniest of children, it will be one of the first keepsakes they place in their scrapbook. For some of the older children, a drawing of themselves will someday help them to realize they were mere children when they arrived at Lily, often without even a name.

These scrapbooks may appear to be a gesture of futility. But I sense God's presence in the midst of it: the books assembled with love by caring women, seeing the children with their own personal scrapbook and the memories they are storing. It is breathtaking for me. Just as the deep rivers carved against mountains and sandy shores of the sea write a story of time and purpose, these books tell a story of lives created by God. Orphaned children are recording their lives here in this place they call home.

Within days of arrival, Katie and I have assembled a list of several nearby children's villages where it is suggested we may find other children who might benefit by having a personal scrapbook. Armed with a scrapbook and directions, we head out to God's Golden Acre, located within a few miles, with a borrowed car from the U.S. couple.

Without specific knowledge of its existence, no one would ever know of the presence of this children's home; it, too, is at the end of a long dirt road. Domesticated dogs happily greet us in the crowded parking lot and an unattended pet pony stands just outside the busy office door. Brennan, a volunteer receptionist, asks how many children I am looking for. I told her 1,000. She laughed, as did I. But I was serious.

Within moments Katie and I explain the use of the scrapbooks by children living at Lily of the Valley and ask if children living at God's Golden Acre would also like to have their own scrapbooks. Myrtle wipes tears from her eyes and says yes as she once again turns the pages of the empty, decorated book. She will arrange for us to return on Sunday to photograph eighty children so their scrapbooks can arrive personalized with their name and photo.

Before we leave she takes us to a large beautiful building with a grand sweeping grass roof that is designed to look like a traditional African building. "This is the theater Oprah [Winfrey] built for God's Golden Acre children. You do know Oprah?" she asks. "Oh yes, we know Oprah," I nod in reply.

The next day Katie and I drive to Richmond, located north by twenty-five miles. We are to meet a woman named Daphne at the roadside near a cemetery. She and her husband Peter Banks moved from a luxurious community of Umlanga (um-shlanga) on the coast to Richmond to open an abandoned baby shelter on an old orchard plot of land they would call eSimphiwe (e-sim-p-way), meaning gift of God. They rely on profits from their swimsuit manufacturing business to sustain them financially and support their dream of this transitional home for babies and young children available for adoption.

Daphne, a strikingly beautiful redhead, takes us to a church-based community center serving people in need with clothing, food, and advice. In an office, I explain to volunteers the use of the scrapbooks by Lily of the Valley children. A woman suggests I go across the street to Bernard Mizeki Primary School, a semi-private school owned by the Anglican Church and the government. Daphne, Katie, and I walk through a gated fence and are greeted by staff watching children on the playground.

We are immediately introduced to the principal, Gillian Bruyns. She invites us into her office and for nearly an hour she tells us the history of Richmond. Having been the principal at this school since before apartheid ended, Gillian describes how anti-apartheid violence between whites and blacks occupied the streets of Richmond. She calls Richmond the epicenter of violence as apartheid began to unravel. The streets were covered with blood spilt during gruesome, murderous rampages. Humans were burned alive—set afire, ringed with car tires, and called "halo of fire." Children sat frozen by fear when stray bullets whizzed overhead through classrooms. Gillian said trembling children would often hide under their desks while she quietly sang a gospel song to comfort them. I explain to Gillian about the scrapbooks being used by children at Lily of the Valley in Mopela. I ask if there are any children at Bernard Mizeki who might benefit by having a scrapbook. Gillian leans toward me with sincere compassion in her eyes and says, "Every last one."

Until today I had only focused on children who had been orphaned. However, Gillian helped me to see that all these children are living with grief and loss due to poverty, violence, and disease. There is no one untouched by the death and destruction in Richmond. Gillian invites us to return to photograph the 260 children attending Bernard Mizeki so each one would receive a scrapbook. Then she graciously invites us for a "spot of tea."

Daphne takes us to a daycare and support center outside of Richmond where children—orphaned or not—come to eat a hot meal of rice and beans. The center serves over 600 local children, however only about 100 children come each day. Katie and I are invited to return next week during a party celebration for Thinabuntu Bahta Desmond's birthday for all children so we can take photographs of the children who will receive a personal memory book. Thinabuntu, a young educated black man, manages the operations and funding of the Richmond Daycare and Support Center with help of twenty local volunteers.

On our way back to Richmond, Daphne takes us to Kwa-Mamuli, a public school where the interim principal has gathered a dozen children who are known orphans to meet with us. We learn the principal of the school has recently died of AIDS. The woman filling in tell us they cannot keep up with staffing due to death and illness related to HIV/AIDS.

As I shake the hand of each student, I notice one young girl unable to look me in the eyes. I follow her gaze to the floor where I see tattered canvas shoes barely covering her small feet. I hold her hand long enough to see her eyes lift to see me smiling. A shy smile emerges briefly. The principal allows us to take photographs of the students so they may receive a scrapbook; Katie records their names on three by five notecards.

Before we leave Richmond, Daphne requests fifty scrapbooks she may use to record a child's earliest days while living at eSimphiwe. She said she would like to send a book with a child to their new home. I am overwhelmed by the ease with which we have found hundreds of children who would benefit by having a personal scrapbook. Daphne treats us to our first encounter with "bunny chow," an Indian meal made of a hollowed loaf of bread filled with curried lamb and vegetables in gravy. Deliciously spicy! Over lunch Daphne reveals she is grieving the loss of her only son. She wonders if loving and caring for orphaned children will heal her own broken heart and once again give purpose to her life.

On the drive to Daphne's home to retrieve our car, Daphne stops by a home where she is aware of a woman who is dying of AIDS. A local social worker has asked Daphne to help convince the woman to take an HIV test so her daughters are eligible for governmental benefits. We enter the cinderblock two-room house where a shadow of a woman is lying on a bed. Filtered sun highlights her hollow face and glassy eyes. Her two teenage daughters are sitting on an adjacent bed with a tiny baby asleep between them. The floor is dirt covered with a small piece of discarded linoleum. The other room has two small tables that hold cooking pots and one small box of potatoes. No stove. No refrigerator. No chairs. No door.

The woman attempts to sit, but trembles and falls back onto the bed. Death is near, but the woman refuses to be tested for HIV due to the stigma of having AIDS. As I leave I notice the attempt at a small garden. The plants are months from yielding food.

In this place, the magnitude of this disaster sweeping across this land becomes real. Everywhere, everyday lives are confronted by disease and death. No one escapes, including the children. Too small to care for themselves, children are victims of abuse and neglect too unimaginable to mention. The thought breaks my heart. The only thing left to do is to pray to God, for in this place God is the only hope that makes any sense. The hope and future of South Africa and the continent of Africa lie in the strength of the remnant left behind: its children. But how will they lead when they themselves have untreated wounds deep within, left from losses most of us never encounter during a lifetime?

During the quiet drive home, I continue to think about the young girl and her tattered shoes; I am reminded of the shame I felt as a child when I, too, wore canvas shoes with holes that revealed my toes. One day at school, Mrs. Hooten, my fifth grade teacher whom I admired, came to school wearing canvas shoes with holes. She taught me that day we are not what we wear. Somewhere inside I felt hope for the child with tattered shoes, that she too would discover the same beautiful lesson through me.

Over the weekend, Noel and Pat invite Katie and me to lunch at a traditional Zulu cultural center. We witnessed the "reading of bones" by a Zulu shaman and tribal dancing accompanied by drums. On Sunday, Katie and I drive through Tala Game Reserve, located directly across the hillside from Lily, where tall giraffes are frequently seen browsing among trees.

Once again Katie and I, armed with directions taken over the phone from South Africans with strong accents, drive north hoping to find additional sites of children's homes in Pietermaritzburg, the capital of the Province of Natal. At SOS Children's Village located in a suburb called

Scottsville, we are let in through a security guard station. I am awestruck at the beautiful brick buildings with white gridded windows surrounded by exquisitely manicured landscaping.

Janine Ward, the manager of this site that cares for 160 children, greets us. The children live in cottages, twelve children with one housemother. On site, SOS offers additional daycare for thirty preschoolers. SOS Children's Village has sister villages around the world; these were first created following World War II by a Swiss businessman in response to the need to care for war orphans.

Katie and I explain the use of the scrapbooks by children living at Lily, and how all other children's villages we have visited, without exception, want scrapbooks for the children they care for. I tell Janine the scrapbooks are a gift to the children without cost to the facility. Janine agrees SOS children need a personal scrapbook to preserve their stories, too. She offers to photograph the children living and attending preschool at SOS and mail their photos directly to us.

With Katie reading sketchy directions, we continue through heavy traffic of Pietermaritzburg and realize after a few turns we are lost. I begin to pray, "God, please help us to find Kenosis Children's Home." Instantly, Katie shouts and points to the sign for Table Mountain. Continuing on, Katie reads we are looking for a road right after a guardrail. As I wonder which guardrail, there it is—a dirt road just past a guardrail. We travel on the road until it turns into a rutted lane through a sugar cane field. Did we miss it? Retracing the way, we see a small stone church steeple nestled under a large grove of trees. Next to the drive we see a small sign for the Lutheran Church, Home of Kenosis Children's Home. Katie and I both sigh. It is quite incredible we are able to find these children's homes that are often at the end of dirt roads appearing to lead nowhere. Each time we arrive successfully, I am more confident as it appears we are simply being led to these homes.

Located in Bishopstowe outside Pietermaritzburg, Kenosis is home to seventeen orphaned children, is sponsored by the Lutheran Church, and is operated by Elke Carrihill and her husband. Elke is touched by the scrapbook concept and offers to put photographs in the books if we send enough for all the children, including her own.

She tells me about a conference being held in Pietermaritzburg in a month that is sponsored by public and private organizations that serve the children of South Africa. "I think you'd enjoy hearing the speakers and networking with people there. Have you heard of the organization that created the Memory Box concept? Parents are encouraged to put together a shoebox of keepsakes the child can keep after the parents die, said Elke.

I knew nothing about the Memory Box, but was curious. Later, when I attended the conference, I met the young man who had created the Memory Box concept. I showed him the scrapbook and began to refer to it as a Memory Book, pointing out how children would use the book following the traumatic loss of parents to re-establish a sense of identity by preserving their own unique story. We each agreed whether memory box or memory book, both appear to be important to the grieving process by children.

Often in the evening after a long day of traveling, Katie and I spend hours back at our cottage on the satellite phone I had rented. The phone requires us to be away from obstructions like trees or buildings so we stand in the middle of the complex. It would be impossible to do that during the day without attracting a crowd of noisy and inquisitive children. So in complete darkness I stand under the stars and talk with Ron about signing up children to receive a Memory Book, or the challenges I face being away. I never want to say good-by, as his voice is both comforting and reassuring.

One hot Sunday afternoon I offer to drive volunteers to the Pavilion Mall in Pinetown. From outside it appears to be domed cathedrals covered with patina copper and glass, but underneath the sub-terrain mall looks like European cobblestone streets. Every few minutes the atmosphere changes from daylight to a starry host overhead. Street lamps running down the walkways light up. It is impossible to tell what time of day it is. Air conditioning keeps shoppers comfortable while escaping from often-unbearable temperatures and humidity outside. I had become so used to the warm climate I buy a sweater just so we can stay long enough to watch a movie in the chilly theater.

In the evenings Katie and I visit the cottages of Lily, and continue to look at scrapbooks with their owners, and help children learn to brush their teeth properly. During the daytime, I visit every single housemother and wash and treat her calloused and worn feet. As I tenderly cradle a housemother's foot over the warm water bath I quietly gasp when I realize this dark skinned foot covered with scars and callouses could resemble the foot of Jesus. A moment I will never ever forget!

One day I spent the entire day ferrying house mothers to voting places in Mopela where each one returns to the vehicle holding up a purple ink stained thumb nail and singing in Zulu all the way home. Each woman professes an unabashed faith in the African National Congress (ANC) candidate. Eugene, a maintenance man and driver at Lily explains that he has been told the ANC is the largest political party and the only one that looks out for the people—people who only recently were given the right to vote. With the size of the ANC, their candidates will most likely always lead South Africa politics.

With only days before we leave Lily, I am invited to come to Pietermaritzburg to visit a children's home housed in an abandoned bus depot. Gail Trollip and her husband and a small staff of people operate Tabitha Ministries. Inside, an assembly line of care giving is underway, preparing babies and toddlers for dinner, bathing, and bed. I offer assistance to help a slippery squirming baby with a bath and diapering. Highchairs line the hallway where toddlers are being fed. A young child with a runny nose cries. I pick him up and hold him in an effort to comfort him—without success. I cradle him close and begin to sway. He sucks on a pacifier and begins to relax. I look into his tear-filled eyes and wonder what he must be thinking. Where is my mother? Early in this trip I remember writing in my journal that God wants the children to know they are loved and he wants to use my arms. I drew his tiny body close to mine and kissed his forehead.

After nearly a month at Lily, Judy returns to pick us up and take us to a volunteer cottage newly opened by the NGO (non-government organization) she and Danie are affiliated with in Hilcrest. Malcolm St. Clair, CEO, arranges for a rented car so we can continue to make visitations to children's homes. Katie suffers being separated from friends she had made at Lily and begins to spend more and more time at the cottage reading. I think she is suffering from culture shock and homesickness.

Just when I think connections for Memory Books may be slowing, more pop up. There is clearly no shortage of orphans, just a shortage of time. Most importantly is to reach those children who are the most vulnerable. When I think of the children who are hungry or starving, alone or afraid, with broken hearts and hopes dashed, I cry out to God and ask that he show me how to find and reach the most vulnerable among them. I read in my devotional Bible about Ruth and her discovery of gleaning of produce from the far edges of the fields. Produce is left in the field because it is too hard to harvest. Her perspective is the value of that which is left is just as valuable in satisfying hunger as that which is easily taken. Large facilities housing orphaned and abandoned children are easy to find just off major roads. But every place God has called us to seems to always be tucked quietly away at the end of a dirt road. People are caring for children quietly and humbly—children who one day may be as instrumental in leading this country as those who always appeared to be destined for it.

Having collected hundreds of requests for Memory Books, I am simply walking and blindly trusting God to provide what is needed to supply children with the message tucked inside a Memory Book that says they are loved by God. I can only hope what I am witnessing will be enough to inspire the hearts of mothers everywhere to assemble these books. I open my Bible and reread the story of God using women to save a child who would one day be called by God to lead his people out of captivity. Would God use one of these children to once again fulfill his purpose in the world? I read of the miracle of Moses' wooden staff turning into a serpent so Pharaoh would know God had sent Moses. A quiet voice said to me, *Tamara, I still use dead wood to perform miracles. What is the Memory Book but dead wood? Throw it down and let me perform a miracle in the midst of a child's story.*

Katie and I travel back to Richmond to photograph as many as 600 children attending Thina's birthday party at the support center. We arrive to find children filling the play yard dressed in what undoubtedly is their finest clothing, often borrowed. Each child is given a 3x5 card on which staff people write their name, sex, and age. When we take the picture we number each card so we can match it with the correct photo.

Looking through the lens of my camera I can see life has been very hard for these children, yet most could manage a fragile smile. Some could not. No child should ever need to wonder how he will eat, where he will sleep, or whether he will be safe or secure or ever be loved again.

After the photos are taken, children enter the large open room inside the center where music and dancing begin the celebration. Thina tells his staff, "All I want for my birthday is to give my children a delicious hot chicken dinner!" Plate after of plate is piled high with curried chicken and rice. Katie and I hand plates to every child. When my hand and the child's hand simultaneously hold the plate, I quietly ask God to bless this child. I often hold the plate an extra long time and wait for the child to look at my smiling face. Though hunger gnaws inside, each child sits quietly and slowly enjoys every single bite of this special gift. As we begin to reach the back of room, my heart sinks as I realize there is not going to be enough to serve everyone. The plates begin to arrive with cold sandwiches; and I grieve as I hand them to the eldest boys in the room.

One child stands to hand me her empty plate and reaches out to hug me. Another child rises and hugs me. Within minutes a line of all the children wait their turn to be hugged. I quietly think to myself, these children must miss the love of their mothers. I continue to hug every single child in line and realize there must be no greater calling then to exchange hunger for life.

Thina pulls Katie and myself to a small room where two plates piled high with curried chicken and rice and eight pieces of chocolate cake await us. I sit starring at the plate of food while a large lump grows in my throat. My thoughts immediately go to the boys who had no chicken. I cannot fathom swallowing any of this delicious food when children went without. Through the window I see the teen boys lined against the fencing and without thought walk toward them with the plate of curried chicken. At first they are confused, but I insist they share it by spoon-feeding each one a scrumptious bite of curried chicken until it is gone. Jokingly catching every morsel escaping from their mouths with the spoon, the boys and I laugh together.

For weeks, Katie and I have traveled throughout these communities to discover hundreds, if not thousands of children living in the wake of a deadly disease. There is no one unaffected by HIV/AIDS where often times there is no one left to mourn. Entire generations of people are simply gone leaving but small children and grannies, the most vulnerable among us. What might the future of this country be, when loss defines every life? What will the world record one day as its response to this great tragedy of widows and orphans?

Chapter 14
Unsung Stories

One day I travel to southern Durban to locate a shelter for abandoned babies called Shepherd's Keep. An attorney, Debbie Wybrow, who works to facilitate adoptions of South African children, suggests I visit this amazing transitional facility. Inside the medical clinic, Cheryl and her husband, who founded the organization, take me to their medical room where I see a tiny premature baby wrapped snuggly in a warm blanket sleeping inside an incubator. The newborn baby boy had been abandoned and brought to Shepherd's Keep. Most other babies are quietly sleeping during their afternoon nap; staff rocked a few on the porch. I arrange to ship generic Memory Books to the facility so they can use them to record events surrounding the child's earliest days while living at Shepherd's Keep.

Katie and I drive down into the valley to Makaphutu (Mock-a-pe-tu) Children's Home. The red metal roofs of the cottages are visible from our own cottage at iThemba. While we wait for permission to photograph the children who will receive Memory Books, a discussion about the arrival of a young local boy is debated among the managers. The young child sits quietly, yet his face filled with fear. Tears have streaked his gray dust-covered face. His mother is known to be dead. His father was arrested recently, leaving the child to walk the streets alone. "When there are known relatives, why should we take him in?" they argue. What must it be like to be alone? Afraid? Hungry and sleepless? Not only unloved, but unwanted as a child? As each child looks into my camera, I see with horror faces resembling death. Washed in gray dust, they often close their eyes in shame and fear of my extended gaze. Oh, how my mother's heart breaks knowing I am unable to comfort them all!

A staff member of Bobbi Bear, an organization that promotes child health following sexual abuse, picks me up one day so I can visit Under the Tree. Under the Tree began when the founder of Bobbi Bear went into a small town and sat under a tree wondering how she could network with community members in enhancing life for women and children. When I arrive I am given an opportunity to explain the use of a Memory Book to store childhood keepsakes and memories. As I photograph each child, it becomes overwhelmingly apparent a Memory Book might appear to be the very least of what these women and children need. Yet, I had to remind myself of what God has given me to give away. I came with neither food, nor clothing, nor money, or an offer of a job. I had nothing but the belief that God could touch and heal the lives of African children through a Memory Book. To those starving or hopeless, this would be a challenge to accept. I am reminded of Noah who built a large boat in the middle of the desert simply because God told him to. Although he suffered ridicule, he remained focused on the vision, not losing sight or commitment. I feel I must do the same. Before I leave here, I have over 100 requests accompanied by photographs of every child present.

After contacting over twenty-five organizations, orphanages, churches, and schools wanting Memory Books for the children they serve, it is hard to understand how anyone would have ill feelings about the Memory Book outreach. One morning, a young man who worked for a local NGO told me the head of his organization had informed everyone who worked for the organization they would be fired if they associated with Memory Books or me. Apparently, a rumor had spread in the community that a woman had taken photographs of African children with the purpose of selling them. I had never been into the valley to photograph children.

Opening an email, I read an article about world-renown author and evangelist Bruce Wilkinson who had developed a multi-faceted outreach in South Africa in which seeds were given to communities so people could grow their own food. A rumor that equated the seeds with the infection of HIV was spread, destroying the entire mission and his reputation. I read with disbelief and wondered if this could also happen to Memory Books. I did not know if this email was a warning or a threat from the sender.

Under a cloak of secrecy, I am meeting with the young man who has been threatened to lose his job if he works with me. He lives in Botha's

Hill, the valley where the rumor had started. He has arranged for me to meet with the unofficial but very powerful leader of the community. I pick up my friend at a Botha's Hill school we had visited earlier in my trip and drove to the woman's home. A young girl answers the door, and invites us to take a seat in the sparsely furnished living room. We sit for 15 minutes while we listen to someone singing in the back of the house. The longer we wait the more anxious I grow. "Tell me about what you are doing," directs a gray-haired black woman who enters the room. I can hardly speak. I pull a Memory Book from my backpack and explain its purpose. I tell her about all the places I have been and the South African people I have had the opportunity to meet.

She takes the book from my hands and slowly turns the empty pages, rubbing her fingers over the playful stickers and attempts to read the captions. "You may continue to do this work. It is good," she finally assures. She explains she is raising her granddaughter after the death of her own daughter. And when her best friend's mother died she, too, came to live here. "I would like to have a Memory Book for my granddaughter and her friend," she says. Overlooking the beautiful green valley, I take photographs of her granddaughter and her friend.

When we drive away, my friend asks me if I know what had just happened. "You will be talked about throughout the valley and will be highly thought of because this woman holds all the power in this valley and will stand up for all you are doing. You need not be afraid of what people try to do to you. She will not permit it," stated my friend. I am humbled to think only God could have orchestrated our meeting. In a place where there is so much about the culture I do not know I could so easily fail. Yet, in this place God is clearly defending and making a way.

Before Katie and I leave South Africa, I meet with Naftaly Ngugi (N-goo-gi), Director of Bambanani (Bam-ba-nah-nee) Camps. He started a camp for disadvantaged and vulnerable children during the summer months. He requests shipment of 100 generic Memory Books the children can use while they attend camp. I also meet with organizers of a Youth For Christ street mission in Pietermaritzburg who hope to use one hundred Memory Books to help children who hope to be reunited with families after being abandoned or running away.

Chapter 15

Another Miracle of Dead Wood

When I arrive home in Oregon, I count the number of requests for Memory Books in South Africa. When I left home, I wondered how I would find 1,000, but to come home with 1,600 requests! Sitting on my study floor I shutter wondering how I am going to fulfill this promise. While it seems overwhelming, there is a part of me that grieves, knowing there are millions of children orphaned in sub-Sahara Africa. But I remind myself, if this is God's idea, there must be a way.

I think about the model my sister Denyce and friend Jennifer designed when the women in their church assembled eighty scrapbooks for Lily children: put together the supplies in a kit for each book, including photographs and names, and ask women to assemble and ship the Memory Books. I began to purchase supplies and invite family and friends to come to my each Monday evening to begin to assemble 1,600 Memory Books. I contact friends throughout the country to request their help. I drive to every Dollar Tree store in the region to purchase every single scrapbook cover in stock. While on business trips, my husband Ron and son Jeff visit Dollar Tree stores, leaving the shelves empty of every single scrapbook cover.

Our basement turns into an assembly line of paper products, plastic sheet covers, and additional pieces for each book that are placed inside a zip-locked pouch and then boxed for each facility. It becomes a time of fun and laughter amongst those of us who are here every Monday. My sister Pamela comes each week bringing along her daughter Alyssa and best friend Lisa and her daughter, Emma. My running friend Stacy shows up religiously and many women from church come as well. Jeff and his wife Holly take turns coming, often bringing Emma, our three-year-old granddaughter to help attach stickers to Memory Book pages.

I receive requests from friends associated with women's groups from all over the country wanting to help assemble and ship these precious gifts for children. Boxes filled with Memory Book kits are shipped to a group of snow birds in Arizona, women in Anaheim Hills, MOPS (Mothers of Preschoolers) groups in Colorado and California, women in transitional housing in Colorado, and a friend of my mother's in Scotland. Women's groups here at home, even nurses I'd once worked with, step up. But still it isn't enough. I have several hundred Memory Books still needing to be assembled and shipped.

I announce within the small group of friends and family that a Monday Night assembly party would begin in the fall, hoping they still had enough enthusiasm to continue to get all the Memory Books fully assembled and shipped to South Africa. I set up an assembly line in our study. On the first night, I sit by myself assembling the Memory Books from the supply kits we had already made. After some time had passed, Ron came in from watching football and sat down. We quietly put together Memory Books, neither of us speaking. But inside I quietly wonder if I am going to fail. Ron asks if I believed God asked me to do this. I had to remind myself of all the times he spoke to me in that quiet yet familiar voice during the past year. In the midst of questionable circumstances I often forget of God's faithfulness. We pray and ask God to show us the way.

Every week the room begins to fill with more and more friends and family who express how rewarding it is to have a part in making this gift for an orphaned child. The house fills with laughter as I get out a toy drum and jokingly implore them to speed up the pace. Quiet conversations of hardships bring solace between friends. The work spills into the dining room and kitchen as more and more people come to help. After two hours of work everything is packed away and carried back into the basement until next Monday. We conclude every evening with dessert and prayer asking God to take this gift and turn it into a miracle, and to heal every child's heart as they wipe away tears with the hankie, just as God's faithful people did in Acts 19.

Many people, including my mother Jean, and Stacy's mother Karen, who are unable to attend Monday Nights offer to hand write letters of hope and encouragement for each child. We place a letter in the back of every single book with a picture of the letter writer.

Each week I make a trip to the post office with boxes and boxes of Memory Books. The postal workers begin to greet me on a first name basis and express amazement at what we are doing. Patrons offer to help carry the precious cargo into the post office. The joy of this simple gesture seems to lift everyone's spirit who takes even a moment to contribute. Amazingly, somehow my checkbook balance always is enough to pay for postage.

I begin to receive emails from various sites in South Africa announcing the arrival of the Memory Books while our group in Gresham, Oregon, is still feverishly assembling and shipping. Our home is cluttered with materials as though an explosion has occurred. Sleepless nights I find myself in the dining room attaching letter stickers spelling out a child's name on the front of the covers. Friends and family agree to come extra days so we can complete every book before the end of the year. On the Monday before Thanksgiving when we place the last book inside a box, everyone present acknowledges the moment with cheers of exhilaration and sheer exhaustion.

Within days of shipping the last of the boxes filled with Memory Books, I receive a large envelop from Malcolm St. Clair in South Africa explaining he had received the contents, but didn't know what to do with it. He thought of the Memory Book and me. Inside I find negatives of children posing individually and a letter from Pastor Elembe Iongwa. "Greetings," he writes. "I am the pastor and director of Group Misa, a refugee camp of Congolese people who have fled the war in our country. We are living inside the Tanzanian border near a town called Kasulu in Kigoma State. The conditions are very extreme as we are not able to leave this place behind fencing. Group Misa is home to several thousand men, women and children grieving because we are unable to return to our homeland because we will certainly face execution." We are looking for help for the people in Group Misa, especially the children. Can you help us?"

What in the world? How is it this comes to me? God, what can I do for these people, I pray. Am I now being asked to provide something more to the people of Africa? How is it that I would know what to offer? Oh God, I am so weary. Can I simply ignore this request?

The quiet, still familiar voice reminds me, *what have I given you to give away?*

It seems too simple, almost ridiculous. *A Memory Book? Can a Memory Book outweigh other needs in value to these children? What if a starving child is handed a Memory Book?* Then I am reminded it is not paper or plastic, but a miracle delivering a message of love. God's love. I think of the time I have spent far away from home facing fear, loneliness, and often, hunger, yet acknowledging all I needed was to know that I am loved by God.

During the past few months, I received other large envelopes from South Africa filled with photographs of children to be inserted in personal Memory Books. I reread Pastor Iongwa's letter and realize he makes no specific request. I ask myself, why wouldn't these children benefit from having their own personal Memory Book. Haven't they, too, lost everything?

On the first Monday night of December Ron and I host a party for sixty friends and family to celebrate what we all have witnessed. Purchasing, assembling, and shipping 1,600 Memory Books to orphaned and vulnerable children in South Africa. We can hardly believe it! Dessert and a prize drawing conclude the evening, except to announce the request of 200 memory books for Tanzania!

Clearly, God is not finished using dead wood!

South Africa

One facility after another, I receive word of the arrival of hundreds of Memory Books after the long four months at sea, rail, and road. Without exception, everyone is excited to begin to record life as it unfolds for a child living in the aftermath of loss. Within weeks, I receive photographs via email and surface mail of children receiving and writing in their Memory Books.

Shortly after, our post office box begins to be stuffed with large envelopes containing thank you letters from children sealed in the self-addressed envelope we placed in a zipper pouch in the back of each book. Often the letters are written on extra paper we had placed in the books. The words of deep appreciation for the Memory Books are so precious, knowing it may indeed be the first and only object that is their only personal possession.

One day I pull a single envelope postmarked from Ontario, Canada, from the post office box. Climbing into my car amidst a rain downpour I read the following words:

Dear Tamara,
My husband and I just adopted an eighteen month-old little boy from South Africa. He was abandoned at birth and rescued by people at Shepherd's Keep outside Durban. Inside a small bag of belongings we found a Memory Book from your organization. It contains photographs, short stories, and comments about the earliest days of our son's life. We wanted to take a moment and thank you for this beautiful gift of preserved memories that would have otherwise been lost forever. It is our hope that one day we will be able to share with our son about his birth and earliest days of life when God rescued him so he could be our son. Thank you so much for giving the staff the idea of recording his life before we knew him. It is an amazing gift.

I re-read the short but absolutely amazing letter again, then place it back inside the envelope and drive home through tears. Until today, I never really expected to see the benefit of a Memory Book by its owner for many years, if ever. After simply walking in blind faith, I felt as though God wanted to assure me I heard Him right. Though a Memory Book may seem too simple, God wants each child living with loss around the world to know: I matter to God. God loves me.

Later that same year, Debbie Wybrow, a South African attorney, won a South African Supreme Court decision to allow adoption of South African children to parents and families outside the country. She emailed me to say she placed a young boy on a plane bound for America. She was so excited to tell me that along with other belongings, she found a Memory Book he would take to his new life in America. "This is amazing work, Tamara!" she wrote.

Chapter 16

The Simplest Word

A sabbatical is how I describe the need to take a few months off before tackling the Tanzania Memory Book request. Even soldiers, often against their will, are pulled from the front lines of battle to rest and recover enough to return to their posts. Pulling back from Memory Books allows me to focus on what I know to be the most important aspect of what God has called upon me to do. All the times I have heard the quiet inaudible voice has been times I am still enough to recognize and acknowledge it. My life has been filled with otherwise good intentions, yet I have often worn myself out by choosing and doing things without asking God if he is still at the helm. Without God, there aren't enough resources in the world to address the human needs around me. Eventually, the focus is on the need and I simply empty myself trying to meet it. After reading from Oswald Chambers devotional book *My Utmost For His Highest*,[10] I write in my journal that when I focus on God and follow him where he is, then I have all the power of God working through me.

It is winter in Oregon. I enjoy the presence of snow flurries since I was in Africa the last two years during the coldest winter months in Oregon. In the quietness of my study, I begin to draft a training manual to use in coordination with Memory Books. It occurred to me the original intent to travel to Africa was to train others in how to help a grieving child. Now that the Memory Book has been developed as a tool for children, surely there will be questions as to how this simple concept will help.

In March, I am invited to a local Christian primary school where third graders will each participate in assembling a Memory Book for a Congolese refugee child. They enclose a handwritten letter about themselves and a photograph. Monday Nights begin and women complete the request of 200 books. One of the Monday Night crew, Sharon Manus, knows the French teacher at the Christian high school and arranges for the French class to write letters in French.

A teacher at Battleground High School in Washington requests I come and invite students to help assemble and ship Memory Books, but cancels the morning of the presentation when I told him I could not leave any reference to God out of the books.

Additional requests from sites in South Africa continue to arrive via email, as many facilities add almost daily to the number of children for whom they care. Dollar Tree scrapbook covers are becoming harder to find, even with the help of the manager in Newberg, Oregon, calling all over the country to no avail. "I'm sorry; there just aren't any more scrapbook covers anywhere in the country," he sighs.

A distant relative, an international scrapbook sales representative, hears about our plight and invites me to attend the national convention in Minneapolis, Minnesota. She contacts the founder of the multi-million dollar organization and arranges for me to meet with her during the convention. As we develop the strategy how to meet the need with the product, the possibilities of what this could mean excite me. "Just imagine," the representative dreamed. "Thousands upon thousands of women purchasing our scrapbook for an orphan!" While praying one day, I hear: Tamara? Will you still love me if I say no? I discounted it, thinking it couldn't possibly be about Minneapolis. It seems to be such a perfect match. I am reminded of my request: if this is you God, bring it to my door.

I fly to Minneapolis. The woman and I drive to the hotel and immediately walk to the convention hall for the first session. Thousands of women and a few men fill the seats while jumbo-tron screens project "highest earner" recipients walking across the stage to receive their awards and rewards: jewelry, lap-top computers, trips, and on and on, all to the screaming approval of fellow sales people. On stage, the founder is introduced to the throng of admirers.

Back at the hotel, I call the cell phone number we had been given to make a time to meet the founder. I leave a message and let her know I am in town. The next day I attend workshops and visit an enormous room displaying products with free samples and discontinued items. Again the day ends inside the convention hall with more rewards and presentations. I quietly think it is so strange I have yet to have a meeting with the founder. Maybe she is going to surprise me and introduce me from the stage, announce a generous donation of scrapbook covers, and we will be able to ship thousands upon thousands of these scrapbooks to orphans. My mind races with crazy ideas.

Arriving back at the hotel with a throng of people jamming the lobby, I recognize the founder near the elevator. "Come," my host says as she pulls on my arm, "there she is!" We push through the crowd. The elevator doors open, she steps on alone while "handlers" hold others back. Then she is gone. My accomplice turns to me and says, "Oh, we were so close."

"What?" I said. "What would we have done if we had reached her? Grab her and introduce ourselves before her security could stop us? 'Oh, excuse me, but I am Tamara Faris and I am the one who wants to talk to you.' All the while her security detail is grabbing us and throwing us to the ground. I can guarantee she would have deemed us as nutcases. Then what?"

As we enter my room, we both sit quietly contemplating what to do next. "I don't think this is it," I said.

"What do you mean? You can't give up this easily," she said. "She is in the same hotel, for heaven sakes. Let's try and call her room," she shook her head as she looked through the presentation she had developed using one of the organization's beautiful scrapbook covers and pages.

"Okay, but this is my last effort. If she doesn't pick up I'll know this isn't it," I reluctantly conceded.

"Hello? Oh, I am looking for . . . "

"Can I ask who's calling?" Said the male voice on the other end.

"I am Tamara Faris from Oregon. I am supposed to have a meeting while I am here."

"Oh. I am her son. She's in the shower. Can I tell her you called?"

"Yes, please."

Alone in my room, I turn out the lights and climb into bed. I cry in the dark. *Why is everything so difficult? What am I doing here? Why isn't this working? Because I'm not in the business of selling scrapbooks,* a quiet yet familiar voice says.

My mind wonders to the euphoria inside the convention hall as sales were celebrated. *What?* I respond. *But, it seems so perfect. Don't you think if God wanted me to meet the founder He could have made it happen. I mean, she is right here in your hotel.* I laugh to myself! She's been here the whole time!

Images of my being pulled through the crowd, trying to catch the founder as she enters the elevator amidst admiring fans and being barred by security begins to makes me smile. What a fool I've been.

Do you still love me? I hear.

What? And then I hear....

Do you still love me if I say no?

Chapter 17

Congolese Refugees

After phone calls from the scrapbook sales representative imploring me to reconsider, I heard that quiet voice say, don't even try and re-open that door. So I set out to design a scrapbook cover myself. When I arrive home from Minneapolis with the door closed by God, I joke with Ron that we would be going into the scrapbook making business to make our own covers. Ron and I fly to Denver to meet with Austin and Jon, sons of our Kilimanjaro friend Rochelle, who started a business called Universal Stylz that imports products from China.

I disassemble a Dollar Tree scrapbook, duplicate all the components, and then set about reassembling it using materials of my choice. Holly helps; my grandchildren, Chase and Emma make painted handprints that ultimately grace our cover. I complete one blue colored scrapbook cover, but assemble a marketing color chart with additional choices in red, green, and yellow tied together with coordinating colored ribbons. We decide to also order the white handkerchiefs as the labor to make our own had grown too labor intensive. We had already worn out two sergers and several seamstresses.

The product sample and color chart and handkerchief design were shipped immediately to China so Universal Stylz could shop for pricing. When the price for the cover comes in at slightly less than two dollars, and the handkerchief at forty-eight cents, we decide to order. The only downside was we had to order at least 10,000 covers and handkerchiefs to get that price. Could we believe God will provide the funds for such a purchase? Could we believe God will help us find enough women to assemble 10,000 Memory Books? Could we afford to ship 10,000

Memory Books? And how long will it take us to find 10,000 children wanting and needing a Memory Book?

My thoughts wonder back to a day when Katie and I sat reading on the front porch of our cottage in South Africa. I had not yet counted the number of requests for Memory Books, and mused myself by thinking how amazing it would be to reach 1,000. Randomly reading through my journal I read passages from Oswald Chambers' *My Utmost for His Highest* I remember to this day. "Why cling to a tiny pinnacle of human endeavor? Why not reach beyond your grasp?"[11] And this quote from Robert Browning's poem, "Ah, but a man's reach should exceed his grasp, or what's a heaven for?"[12]

If I were to live my entire life for others, I think, what regret would there be in that? If it takes the rest of my life to ship 10,000 Memory Books, what else would be more rewarding?

By now I am accepting every offer to speak to anyone who will take the time to listen to the story about Memory Books. I am invited to speak to large groups and small groups; those who need no arm-twisting in believing, and some who are quite skeptical.

By the insistence of my mother Jean, I agree to speak to a local Rotary Club attended by one of her neighbors. "This is a pretty rough group," he warns me. "Their really interested in local things for which they get a lot of publicity." I manage to overcome the interruptions of latecomers and servers delivering breakfast croissant sandwiches. I finish a very brief overview of the Memory Book project and ask if there are questions. Sitting in the front seat, a white haired gentleman sat with arms crossed over his chest, questions, "Tell me what good is a scrapbook to an orphan. Aren't there plenty of other things they need more?"

"That is a very good question," I reply. Inside I thought, *yes, that is a very good question. What is the answer? God, what is the answer?* I began to speak slowly hoping an answer would arrive on my lips. "Sir, say you've just had the worst day of your life. You've lost your job. You've come home to find your wife has left you. Your dog has run off. Your entire life has collapsed and you have lost everything. When you arrive home you go to the mailbox."

A man interrupts, "And the IRS says you owe them millions!" The room erupts in laughter. I sense I'm losing them. This has become a joke to them.

God, I pray, *help me make the point.* "You go to the mailbox, here on the worst day of your life, and reach in and pull out a single letter. Inside it reads, 'You do not know me. I live on the other side of the world. God asked me to tell you that He loves you so much. Here, today, on the worst day of your life, God is near. He never will leave you. He sees your tears. He knows your broken heart. He hears you when you pray. God loves you.' Tell me, sir just how amazing would that be?" I repeat, "Just how amazing would that be? That's the message that comes in every Memory Book, sir."

For months I continue to work on the training manual. Stacy and I develop the concept of children having a club setting so they can work on their Memory Books. In one afternoon I write a complete format for facilities to host a monthly Memory Book Club, including theme songs, a talking stick, and lessons about identity, self-esteem, purpose in life, and remembering those I love, all accompanied by a craft.

The purpose of the Memory Book Club is to give children an opportunity to tell their own unique story in the midst of loss while having a witness. I learn how to buy a music license so we can include music and words in all 250 first edition copies of our training manual. Joan Schweitzer Hoff, Director of Program Development at The Dougy Center for Grieving Children and Families,[13] offers to edit the chapters related to child grief and loss. Joan praised the Memory Book Club concept as it follows a similar approach of peer support groups used successfully at The Dougy Center.

As the Memory Book Club concept continues to develop among women attending Monday Nights, several women suggest we go to South Africa and introduce Memory Book Club in person to sites where children already have Memory Books. Just as the previous year, a vision for the coming year is revealed just before we conclude the year.

Again, Ron and I host what is now the Annual Celebration of Memory Books in the hands of South African orphans and Congolese refugees in Tanzania. I thumb through the guest book everyone signs each Monday Night and discover hundreds upon hundreds of hours spent by over sixty women, men, and children investing in the lives of children on the other side of the world. I recount the instances of God's faithfulness to support all we need, but also include the times I had to learn of his ways the hard way. The evening ends with the drawing for prizes from names of those attending each Monday Night; the drawing is a simple way to thank those who have given so much of their time.

Tanzania

With news of the elimination of surface shipping to Africa, I fear shipping boxes of memory books by air to Tanzania would make it cost prohibitive. The clerk at the post office counter said, "These are books, right? Why aren't you shipping them in an M-bag? The books will be shipped air in half the time, and it is even cheaper than surface once was."

As I drove to the post office that day, the dread of the Memory Books not arriving in time for children dying of disease weighed heavy, yet I had no idea how we could afford to ship by airmail instead of surface mail. Now I find out that not only were the Memory Books going to arrive in two to three weeks, but also shipping costs were cheaper using book rates in an M-bag. It may sound cliché, but when a door closes, I simply find another door.

After the boxes were mailed, I had visions of them traveling their final journey bouncing in the back of a truck, the dust of the tires visible for miles across the desert plain of Tanzania. I imagined the pastor requesting permission to pass through numerous security check-points as he made his way back to the refugee camp outside the town of Kasulu with boxes of Memory Books carried by an ox cart. I thought of the curious look by desperate refugees when scrapbooks were unpacked and distributed among the children. Within weeks I receive word via email from Pastor Iongwa and General Secretary Abwe Innocent of the Memory Books' arrival at the refugee camp. What an amazing accomplishment! This small gift to the children of Group Misa, halfway around the world from my home! They have arrived!

Within weeks I receive a large envelope covered with literally dozens of stamps. Inside the negatives of photographs of children receiving their personal Memory Books. One photo shows a young girl holding a Memory Book by the ribbon tie, and our family Christmas family photo I had placed in a Memory Book clearly visible while tucked inside the belt of her pink dress.

During the coming months, we begin to receive padded envelopes of thank you letters from French speaking children at Group Misa that were translated into English by adults. All the letters extend deep appreciation for the Memory Book and request prayer for the desperate situations they are living in as refugees. An accompanying letter from Pastor Iongwa says several thousand men, women, and children are not allowed to leave the fenced area along the border with their homeland. Food and shelter are limited. The threat of having to return to their homeland by Tanzanian officials would certainly result in their execution by the rebels.

Many of the hundreds of thank you letters from Group Misa are addressed to children at Portland Christian School, a church in Stevenson, Washington, and a home school group in Skamania, Washington, to name a few. I attempt to forward them with a request to continue to correspond with each child.

During the holidays, our Monday Night group collects new soccer balls, jump ropes, small stuffed animals, and toy cars and ships four large boxes of gifts to Group Misa, Congolese refugee children.

Chapter 18
Unexpected Ending

"Excuse me?" I respond.

"I'm sorry, but I cannot let you board the plane. Your passport does not have enough blank pages to accommodate the size of the South African immigration stamp."

"That is impossible. Let me see." The South African Airlines official hands me my passport and I flip through the pages in an attempt to correct him. There in the middle of the last two empty pages was a small immigration stamp from my recent trip to Australia with my mother. Why in the world would immigration in Australia use a completely empty page for their tiny stamp?

"Sir, is there anyway I can still board? You don't understand. I am leading a group of people to South Africa including many who are traveling abroad for the first time."

"If I let you make the flight, immigration in South Africa will simply put you back on the next flight. You can layover in here and visit the US Immigration Office in downtown Washington, D.C., where they can sew additional pages into your passport while you wait. We can put you on the flight to South Africa tomorrow night."

I cannot believe this is happening. Neither can Stacy, Andrea, Doranna, and Bryan when I describe what I have to do. What they have to do.

"Stacy, I am going to give you my trip planner. Remember when you get to Johannesburg you'll have to take your luggage from the international terminal and walk up the street to the domestic terminal. Locate South African Airways counter where they'll put the luggage on the domestic flight. When you are walking up the sidewalk, don't let anyone help you with your luggage, even your backpack. Wear your backpack on the front. Thieves can pilfer through your pack without you even knowing it. When you get to Durban, Malcolm and Beverly will be waiting for you. Go to the rental agency where I've reserved a twelve-passenger van."

Stacy is calm, but I know she is terrified with the thought of driving in South Africa. "You can do this, Stac. I have all the faith in the world you can do this." We pray together before they leave the gate to board the plane without me.

As the gate empties, I meet a young couple from Chicago. They are on their honeymoon and have encountered the same situation. And I thought my circumstances were dreadful! The beautiful young woman travels internationally a great deal for business, and, unfortunately, was not aware her passport didn't have enough space. Taking pity on me, the husband invites me to share a cab to downtown Washington, D.C., hotel just blocks from the immigration office. After checking in they invite me to join them for dinner.

The place is jammed with people still wearing business attire, but obviously no business is being done on this Friday night. The three of us stand awkwardly quiet waiting for a table in the midst of deafening conversations. After ordering, I laugh out loud to them saying, "I bet you never dreamt you'd be having dinner with a complete stranger on the first night of your honeymoon. "

In the morning in the midst of drizzling rain, we meet to walk the five blocks to the immigration office that opens at 9 a.m. Because of traveling needs of politicians and diplomats, it is the only immigration office in the country that attaches additional pages inside your passport while you wait. While we wait the two hours, I learn he is a physician completing his surgical residency in Chicago. When he is done, they would like to move somewhere warm like San Diego. They had thought about Oregon. It is a beautiful place to raise a family, I say, but I'm not sure the weather can be defined as warm.

That evening we board the flight to Johannesburg. In the dark cabin somewhere over the Atlantic Ocean I try to make sense of what just happened. In so many ways, God has resolved dilemmas over and over again. Why not this time? I laugh to myself when I think about the story this couple will tell.

I realize we had become friends as we helped one another overcome the dilemma we faced together. Laughing about our circumstances, at the same time being grateful it was so easily resolved. I wonder to myself: If I am never to see them again, what could I say that would make these twenty-four hours worth the inconvenience? What could I share with this newly married couple? I knew immediately, yet wondered how I'd say it.

Waiting for our luggage, I tell them I think that we were meant to meet. "Really?" they inquire.

"My husband and I have been as much in love as the day we were married thirty-five years ago," I said. "I want to tell you how we stay married. But promise me this one thing. Even if you don't believe it now, when and if the day ever comes you are ready to give up on your marriage, remember the day we met and give some thought to what I am sharing with you. I think we met because I am supposed to tell you to make God first in your lives together. That's what has been our solid foundation and common denominator. That's the answer." Their reaction isn't unexpected because I think they've come to realize this whole thing has been crazy.

"After retrieving our luggage," he says, "if your flight is delayed or cancelled, we'll be staying at the hotel here before our flight to Port Elizabeth tomorrow. Call us. We can have dinner."

"Oh, sure!" I retort, laughing out loud. "I can just picture the scene of my calling. You answer the phone in your room, place your hand over the receiver and tell your wife, 'OH MY GOSH! It's her again! She's here at the hotel! What do I tell her? What do we do?'" We hug amidst laughter, and I thank them and wish them a wonderful honeymoon and life together, acknowledging that sometimes friendship is for a moment.

It is Sunday evening. Malcolm has the traditional Sunday braai of chicken on the barbeque. I am so relieved we have all arrived in South Africa safely and mostly unscathed by the ordeal. The two stories of our separate journeys finally merge here with great laughter and amazement as we each tell our own version. Months ago, Malcolm and Beverly graciously accepted my request to house the five of us over the next two weeks in their beautiful home situated under grand cypress trees defining the town of Kloof. I had already learned to value the opportunity to separate myself from the work while in South Africa. It was my hope to help balance the work we were about to begin with relaxation for my friends.

Over the past several months, Stacy, Andrea, and Doranna have organized the supplies needed to introduce the Memory Book Club to the children's homes. Here in South Africa, Debbie Morgan has created art supply buckets filled with crayons, paint with brushes, scissors, colored pencils, hole punches, and cleaning supplies for each facility we plan to visit. Andrea has brought twenty handmade crocheted baby blankets with newborn clothing and a small toy she calls Baby Bundles. Bryan, a photographer I met while volunteering at a foster kids camp, offered to come on this trip to help document the trip with photos. While much of the schedule is pre-planned, there is plenty of time we will simply go where we are led.

Monday morning we load the van with everything needed to host a Memory Book Club. We leave the town of Kloof for the familiar drive to Lily of the Valley outside Mopela, forty-five minutes away. As I turn onto the dirt road leading to Lily, I see a small block building under construction where a medical clinic is planned. It was the last request of Marion, the nurse I first met at Lily four years ago, before she died of cancer. Under shade trees I see women sitting together beading in front of the community center dedicated the year Katie and I were here. More vegetable tunnels are erected; the building housing a community day care (crèche) looks inhabited with curtains billowing from the open windows. As I pass the volunteer house built for the U.S. couple and their children, I notice a tall fence with padlocked gate encircling an overgrown, abandoned site.

Just as Lily of the Valley has grown, so indeed have the children. Upon climbing from the van I immediately recognize a young girl, yet much older, as one I had treated in the clinic for fever and flu symptoms during my very first visit to Lily four years ago. We are greeted by the social worker that had arranged our visit. As we are discussing the format for Memory Book Club, I hear a wail behind us. It is Big Martha running toward me wailing my name, her arms waving. When we meet, she grabs my neck and we embrace. "Ta-mar-ah!" she cries. "God has brought back my dear friend, Ta-mar-ah!" I remembered when we parted two years ago; she sobbed when I left, "Why does God take away a friend, just when he gives me a friend?" At that time, I had no idea whether I would ever again see Big Martha or anyone who called Lily their home.

With preschoolers already assembled in the classroom, the four of us try to teach the children how to sing "I Am Somebody" while Bryan takes photographs.

> I am somebody, I am somebody.
> And I know that my worth is not found on this earth.
> I'm a child of the Most High God.
> (author unknown)

None of us are very good at singing; fortunately, these grateful children don't care.

Making the crown craft for preschoolers is lots of fun, especially squeezing the white glue tube! We end up with lots of glue everywhere. But when we tie the crowns upon their heads, no one cares about anything but the images Bryan captures with his camera. We end Memory Book Club by trying to sing a song about God knowing our name. Even when following the words on a card, we still don't get it right, but the children don't care. They simply beam beneath their crowns.

When children arrive home from school shortly after lunch, we hold another Memory Book Club for that age group, duplicating our earlier efforts with the same moving moments as we announce their names as we "crown" them royalty, heirs to God's kingdom. When we ask if any of the high school children will join us singing, they all jump up, leaving no one as an audience.

Each day that follows we load the vehicle and head off for yet another site where Memory Books have been placed. On the day we plan to go to Mother of Peace, we stop at Under the Tree where several dozen women are singing. I look among their faces and see no one I recognize. I explain I came two years ago and distributed Memory Books among the women for their children, but still no one understands why we are here. Years ago, I remember a woman driving up to the tree in a black Mercedes, getting out, and opening the trunk of her car to reveal loaves of day–old mangled bread. The women formed a line and when the bread was placed in their hands, they each walked away holding it so carefully you would have thought it was a priceless artifact.

I pray and plead silently, *God, what do I have to give these women?* Stacy retrieves my Bible from the car and a young woman offers to translate. I share the devotion I had read earlier that morning that stated the Lord is the bread of life and he is all we need. When I finish the women begin to sing in Zulu. The four of us sit among them, hold their babies, even dance when they insist we join them. Then the young girl who translated turned to me and said, "But the women are still hungry. These woman have nothing to eat."

Stunned, I ask God again, *what do I have to give away?* I walked to the trunk of our car and pull from the cooler and basket the exquisite lunch we had prepared for the five of us to enjoy while at Mother of Peace. Sandwiches of salmon pate, cucumbers, and baby lettuce layered between beautifully sliced bread; fresh fruit, crackers, cookies, and even hot water for powdered chai tea lattes. I lay the entire meal out on a blanket; the young girl begins to cut it up into tiny servings, handing each woman a morsel to taste. At the end of an unplanned day of fasting and putting on Memory Book Club for Mother of Peace children, the five of us each filled the empty pit in our stomach with a cup of chai tea at the back of the car, enjoying every drop. Unlike the women under the tree, we know we will never have to worry about when we would eat again.

One day, we travel to God's Golden Acre and host Memory Book Club for dozens of children. It rains so hard the noise on the metal roof makes it impossible for the children to hear a word we say or sing. The harder it rains the harder everyone laughs. Almost the entire group of children wearing their just-made crowns joins us on the stage while we again attempt to sing. Myrtle explains that many of the older girls had been moved to Oprah's new school for girls. I look into the eyes of those young teen girls who had been left behind and wonder how painful it must be to not be chosen. I think of my holey canvas shoes and Mrs. Hooten and quietly hope these beautiful girls will learn their value comes from who God says they are, and not from what others think. Their lives hold promise and purpose. My life is testimony to that.

We travel north to Pietermaritzburg to visit SOS Children's Village where we learn the facility has a new manager who had found unused Memory Books stored in a closet. When visiting one of the cottages, a housemother knows of the Memory Books and explains that yes, the children have them and are using them.

Visiting Bernard Mizeki Primary School, we find Memory Books stacked on shelves in every classroom and used as part of the curriculum. Armed with crown kits containing crowns cut from paper plates, plastic jewels, black yarn ties, and glue, we visit every classroom. The 260 children are so excited to show us their personal Memory Books filled with precious keepsakes and memories. After lunch with staff, we watch weak-kneed as the children fill the entire play area and sing for us as they all wear their crowns.

During breakfast the next morning, Bryan remarked, "Do you know Casting Crowns [a Christian rock band]? That is what we are doing." Stacy and I run out into a morning downpour of rain and dance with joy of the thought that we are truly casting crowns!

On the day we visit Sinikithemba Clinic at McCord Hospital, Dr. Holst's personal assistant takes us on a tour of the hospital. Andrea, Stacy, and Doranna visit the Labor and Delivery Unit where they give new mothers a gift for her baby. Doranna meets a young mother who had delivered a baby with Down Syndrome and was able to encourage her by her own experience of adopting two children with Down's Syndrome. A social worker invites us to join her as she visits a school in Adam's Mission where she is using the Memory Books in an after school program. She takes us to a home where a woman is caring for a dozen orphaned girls, and her brother is caring for young boys in a house next door. When we arrive, the teenagers all bring their Memory Books and we spend the next hour looking through the pages with them. One young girl pulls a neatly folded letter from the page titled "Letters I Write." She begins to read the letter she had written to God that contains every single detail from the day her mother died; she ends her letter by thanking God she and her brother are still alive even though all their relatives are dead.

We arrange to return to Adam's Mission to visit another site where three women and one man are caring for about twenty-five children orphaned in their neighborhood. We sit on a cement floor with the children as they decorate their crowns. One young girl takes Stacy into her room and shares the tremendous grief she is living with.

Every single day is difficult to face, yet this day seems the hardest. Compared to Lily, Mother of Peace, SOS, or God's Golden Acre, these children and adults are barely getting by. When we leave here we are all prompted to do something more, so we arrange for Debbie Morgan and Malcolm to purchase and deliver small plastic tables and chairs so the children will have someplace to eat and do homework other than the cold, hard, cement floor.

By the end of the second week, everyone is absolutely exhausted physically and emotionally. At dinner, I comment I am concerned whether the group has enough strength and bravery to continue through the rest of the week. I let them know it will only get harder, and question whether they feel they can travel north where it will be even more challenging. "Because," I hesitated, "WE ARE GOING ON A SAFARI!" I jump from my chair, and they all just look at me in stunned silence.

"What?" they ask.

"We are going on a safari. We leave tomorrow and will drive north to Phinda where we'll stay for three days." The safari is a surprise and gift from Ron and me for the group because of their dedication to Memory Books to the extent of taking the risk to come to Africa. Besides, Ron and I just love surprising people when we can, and I knew these helpers would need a good uplifting adventure.

Before bed Doranna receives devastating news her daughter's father-in-law had died. While away, life continues at home, taking good and bad turns for each of us. It helps remind me that while we can take a moment to enjoy Africa's beautiful bush land and its inhabitants, life is fragile.

The next morning the five of us load the van for the drive to the game reserve. Along with our own personal items, we bring one art supply bucket we have yet to give away and two sets of Andrea's Baby Bundles. This will be my fourth trip to Phinda Private Game Reserve, owned and operated by Conservation Corporation Africa (CCA), which is dedicated to returning land once farmed to its natural bush land state. Phinda (meaning 'the return' in Zulu) has won awards for responsible, sustainable ecotourism, and empowering and enriching local communities with employment, infrastructure, and micro-business loans.

As I drive for four hours north on N2 toward Richard's Bay and then on to Phinda, we all began to relax and lose ourselves in the beauty of the surrounding landscape. It feels so good to know of the reward Phinda would be after all the difficult days we have had visiting places where deep loss defines life. I stop and pay at the tollgate, and know the next stop will be to exit the freeway toward the small game reserve of Phinda.

Within moments I have to slow for two men dressed in beige uniforms standing along side the freeway motioning us to stop. After years of driving in South Africa I know to not pull over for anyone and made the decision to continue. From the car's side mirror I see two cars racing toward us. One car pulls in front of me while the other car's driver motions for me to pull over. The slowing car in front forces me to slow while the other car swerves toward me, forcing me to the shoulder. With both unmarked cars parked fifty feet ahead, a black man dressed in the beige uniform   walks toward our car while another black man in the same uniform stands behind their vehicles.

I roll down the window. In very broken English the man demands my driver's license. He impatiently motions for me to get out of the car and follow him. "I must arrest you for fleeing our check point!" he angrily shook his finger at me. He opened the trunk of his car, and shouted, "I am arresting you!"

"What? I'm sorry, sir. I didn't recognize you as police. I saw no badging to distinguish you as police officers." Under direct sun, beads of sweat covered his forehead and large veins bulged from the sides of his neck. His eyes filled with red anger.

"I am arresting you. You must come to the police station to pay the fine." He reached into the trunk of the car and pulled out a white three ring binder. Flipping through the pages listing infractions, he points to the fine for fleeing, which is 1,000 Rand (about 140 dollars in U.S. currency). Both men speak to one another in Zulu.

Initially, I simply want to do what is required and get on with the day. "How long will this take, sir? I do not have time as I am taking a group of American friends north for an appointment later today," I said.

"You must come to the police station to pay the fine," he shouts.

Something inside me tells me something is not right. I begin to pray silently. Inside the trunk, I see there are ropes and chains. Inside my chest my heartbeat begins to accelerate. Not wanting the men to see my fear, I attempt to slow my breathing while something inside me is screaming: this is not what it appears to be! Something is telling me that even if they take me to the police station I will not be safe. And worse, what if I never make it to the police station? Something inside me says: whatever I do, don't go with these men. For a split second I think it may be less dangerous to run into the street and attempt to stop someone than to go with them.

"Sir," I said, "I am so sorry. I didn't know you were a police officer." Hoping to ingratiate him, I said, "My son is a police officer in Oregon. I would never ever do anything against the law. Please, is there anything I can do right here to make this right?"

"No! You must come to the station to pay the fine!" He is becoming increasingly adamant.

"Please, sir, can I just pay the fine here right now?" Inside, I am begging God to help me.

Again, the angry man emphatically states, "You must come to the station to pay the fine." I wonder how much more resistance this man will tolerate. Again, the two men speak to one another in Zulu, and appear to argue. The quieter of the two turns his back to us.

Please, I quietly plead.

"Is there anyone in your car who can drive?" he asks.

"No, I am the only one licensed to drive the rental vehicle." I sense he is attempting to make it possible to separate me from my friends. I look up to see Bryan has exited our van and is walking toward us. *Is there anyone who can drive?* keeps repeating itself in my head. *No. No, there is no one who can drive. No. No, there isn't,* I say to myself. As Bryan gets closer I look into his eyes with a deep and pleading look, hoping he will hear my inaudible plea. *Say no, Bryan. Say no. Say no, Bryan. Say I am the only one who can drive.*

As Bryan gets closer I see he is looking into my eyes. Pleading inside, *say no, Bryan.*

"Can you drive that car?" the man asks Bryan. Bryan looks away to the man.

"No. I am not insured to drive the vehicle," he says confidently. "Only she can drive it," he points to me.

"Sir?" Bryan said. "I am so sorry we have violated your local laws. We are visiting from America, working with the orphans in your communities. I am so sorry we have inconvenienced you."

The men speak to one another in Zulu. "Five hundred rand," the angrier man barks. "You must pay a fine of five hundred rand."

"Bryan, go get five hundred rand from my purse," I said.

"But?" Bryan attempts to question why.

"Bryan," I repeat, "go get five hundred rand from my purse." I feel a sense of urgency knowing these men could very well change their mind if they sense we are arguing with them. Bryan finds five hundred rand neatly folded inside my wallet placed there this morning for our drive north. The only money I have. I place the neatly folded bills into the man's hand. As he closes his fingers around it, I realize inside that these men are either corrupt police officers or simply dressed to scam motorists or worse. Either way, seventy dollars may not seem like a lot of money, but it very well could be the cost of life today.

With my driver's license in my hand, I turn and begin to put one foot in front of the other. I fear I will feel the hands of one of them grip my shoulders with a change of heart. My legs feel paralyzed; I fear I will collapse or the men will reconsider before I am able to reach the van. Once inside, my legs struggle to operate the manual transmission as I pull away from the scene. Doranna, Andrea, and Stacy are still praying. Bryan is recounting his role in the event. I am simply thanking God under my breath.

I relax knowing God has already taken care of the highlights my friends will enjoy while at Phinda. We all laugh when greeted by a roaming giraffe at the front gate. The impromptu British style tea alongside an elephant watering hole. All of God's creation is on parade. From cheetahs, to rhinoceros, wart hogs, varieties of antelope, springbok and dikas, monkeys and lions. Swimming across the pool, Stacy is introduced to the water scorpion. "Yuck!" we scream, deciding we would simply enjoy the pool from our chaise.

We enjoy the lantern lit dinner, but my favorite surprise is the champagne breakfast at the hippo swamp. That morning the game ranger, Cooper, explains he is from Zimbabwe. He fled his homeland with his mother and brother after military officials killed his father and pet dog when he refused to turn over their farm for reclamation of land back to Black Zimbabweans. Cooper shows us a female lion with three cubs. One has fallen ill and struggles to keep up with the mother and siblings. It is extremely painful to watch the female lion grapple with the dilemma of leaving her cub behind so she can hunt. With one last glance, she climbs through the briars where the other two cubs wait for her. While veterinary skills would certainly benefit the dying cub, Phinda is dedicated to allowing the life cycle to fulfill itself. We simply become a witness to nature. Doranna is overwhelmed by the loss and writes a beautiful epitaph of the little cub's short life in Phinda's guest book.

While I refuse to let the safari be ruined for my friends by what happened on the way there, the remnants of fear that had settled inside me stir without warning. The "what ifs" keep attempting to paint a picture of dread in my thoughts. God's magnificent creation around me helps to push them aside temporarily. I don't feel I know fully what had happened, so I resolve to underestimate what could have happened.

Before leaving Phinda, we offer the art supply bucket to Cooper who will give it to the local school children. Stacy gives Cooper a leather-bound copy of Oswald Chambers devotional *My Utmost for His Highest*, which she treasures for its daily inspiration. While passing women carrying babies on the road, Andrea decides to stop and simply hand a Baby Bundle to the surprised mother. I enjoy the look on their faces from the rear view mirror as we drive away.

Chapter 19

Stories Without Words

We fly to Johannesburg together, but my friends will fly home to the USA without me. In Johannesburg I plan to meet Joan Schweitzer Hoff from The Dougy Center; we will fly to Rwanda together. Bruce and Anita Paden, World Venture missionaries living in Goma, Democratic Republic of the Congo for the last twenty years, opened a center for grieving children in Goma. They have invited us to come conduct training on child grief and loss for twenty-five school principals, and introduce them to the use of Memory Books to help children tell their story in the midst of loss.

Outside the plane, enormous thunderheads are mushrooming from the African plains below as multiple flashes of lightning illuminate the edges. Inside the darkened plane most travelers are sleeping, including an exhausted Joan. I wonder how anyone can sleep through the rattling turbulence. The sky ahead is black against remnants of a setting sun. Suddenly, a bright light fully engulfs the plane, and again my heart races and panic sweeps over me. Why is everyone asleep? The plane immediately turns steeply to the right, then immediately turns steeply to the left as though we are flying through an obstacle course of lightning bolts. There are no typical announcements of turbulence coming from the cockpit. I feel like I'm in a bad dream and anxiously wonder if this is how disastrous crashes begin.

After an overnight stay in Kigali, Bruce and Anita drive Joan and me over the mountain range to the Rwanda border town of Gisneyi where we will cross into The Congo and the city of Goma. Even Bruce and Anita choose to fly into Kigali and drive to Goma because airlines flying into the Congo are too dangerous, often using retired Russian planes. The evidence of crashes lies crumpled at the end of the Goma runway.

The border crossing is one right out of the movies. Hundreds of people are pressing against a window being served by a slow and disinterested official. Bruce and Anita lead us through an open door guarded by armed military. A man wearing reflective sunglasses rises from behind a desk and shakes Bruce's hand. Several other uniformed officials are seated at desks. We are offered a place to sit while Bruce fills out visa forms for us. Within minutes we are walking toward a gate over the road while others are still fighting for attention at the window.

There may not be another place on earth exactly like Goma. It is as if civilization has left it behind. As the jeep shakes and rumbles across the hardened molten lava streets, Anita tells us about a recent eruption of the volcano looming over the city. The volcano is one of only two open calderas in the world where hot molten lava lights the sky pink at night. Apparently the lava flowed down the mountainside, terrorizing everyone. But, it suddenly disappeared into a large fissure in the earth leaving everyone relieved. Life returned to normal, but suddenly hot molten lava began to come up from the ground right in town, destroying everything in its path. The lava flowed down the streets and into Lake Kivu. The heat from the lava killed aquatic life including fish and plants that were close to the area where the lava spilled into the lake. Lake Kivu has the reputation of being the gassiest lake in the world. It contains cubic kilometers of methane and carbon dioxide gas. People and animals have been known to suffocate from gas that has collected in the pockets on the surface of the lake. With a towering inferno overhead and a lake of deadly water, Goma feels more like an imaginary place in a horror film than a real location. When Bruce learns Ron and I climbed Kilimanjaro he tells me, "People used to be able to climb the volcano, until a Chinese lady fell into the caldera." I shuttered with the thought. "Climbing Nyiragongo is also dangerous because of rebel groups that now operate near the mountain," Bruce adds.

"Don't touch the walls inside the shower," Anita tells me as we settle into our rooms. "We have stray electricity going through the walls and we can't seem to resolve it." The house overlooks the lake, a lovely setting had I not known the waters were deadly. Surrounding the house is a ten-foot tall rock wall, manicured grass, and lovely flower-filled beds. The covered front porch has a large conference style table and chairs, and on the side of the house a porch swing overlooks the lake. Next door, a vacation home for the Governor of the State is always guarded by the military. Bruce tells us they feel safer knowing government officials live close by.

After a light dinner of spaghetti, chicken, bread, and hot tea I am ready to crash into bed. Bruce asks that we lay clothes out and keep our backpacks with passports ready to go if the rebel forces come close to the house. He tells us that the rebels are north now so it should remain calm. In my darkened room, I change for bed; outside the window I watch as a young man operates his business selling phone minutes from inside a dimly lit wooden building the size of small school bus shelter.

The next morning we drive through town where a bustling market lines the streets. People are coming and going. Without warning I see a hatchet rise and fall across the neck of a chicken on a stump and a dead goat for sale hanging in a tree. Rarely is anything packaged like the way Americans buy shoes or food, and a haircut or shave may be done as everyone looks on. "Can we go to the main part of town, Bruce?" I ask.

"This is it," he laughs.

Some parts of the city have been rebuilt since the eruption, but many businesses are abandoned. Life simply started over when the molten rock cooled and hardened. The traffic slows; beside the jeep I watch as a regiment of police officers march by, jabbing guns with bayonet's, spears, and large hatchets in unison with each step. Bruce says it is a show of intimidation for anyone who might think of breaking the law.

We drive to New Hope Center, a place for children experiencing loss and grief that was opened and funded by Bruce and Anita. Fitina operates the center that sees several hundred children per year. Within the compound, a European NGO shares space to operate a training center for teenage boys and girls. Joan and I survey the setting for the two-day training that begins tomorrow. Before we leave I have an opportunity to invite the children at the center to draw a picture using paper and crayons I brought. Then the children play drums while we parade around the room.

The principals, mostly men, represent 25,000 children attending schools in the surrounding area. Most attendees have traveled overnight to attend the seminar at The Hope Center. My experience with seminars in Africa is people expect to be paid to come, including housing, transportation, and meals. Bruce and Anita have found funding in their meager budget; this training is that important to them. The training begins with introductions as Bruce interprets French into English for the two of us. Joan spends the morning defining mourning and grief using examples of how loss produces external and internal responses.

Outside the building I hear vehicles and honking at the gate. Everyone goes to the windows and doors to watch as United Nations' peacekeeping military jeeps enter the compound. Uniformed men with light blue berets or turbines stand in the back; they are armed with automatic weapons. From one of the many vehicles climbs a man dressed in a pristine, yet limp, white shirt and slacks, accompanied by several U.N. officials. Having exited the building with my camera still in hand, I slowly tuck it behind my back in fear I would be accused of taking their photographs. Bruce meets with the men and informs us it is a Swiss government official wanting to visit the training center next door.

When lunch is served, everyone comes to the tables with plates piled so high with food that some often falls from the plate. Anita tells us this may be the only meal they eat for some time, evident by the slight frame of most Congolese.

After a long morning of theory and an enormous lunch, I worry everyone will fall asleep at their tables when my presentation begins. Without explaining, I begin to sing "I Am Somebody." While my singing may not have improved much since the song's début in South Africa earlier, I attempt to teach them the song amidst much laughter. I explain the concept of using a Memory Book for children to draw or tell their story when words are too difficult or language has not yet formed for younger children.

I pass around the crown kit as an example of crafts the children can make when they attend a Memory Book Club. As I am talking, I notice each man is taking a paper plate crown, ties, and jewels from the kit and laying it on the table in front of them. I realize they want to make a crown themselves. Colored pencils are distributed and for the next hour, grown men are designing beautifully decorated crowns with their names. I offer to tie a man's crown when I realize he wants to wear it, but struggles to tie it. One after another, they come to have me tie their crowns, a gesture I have done literally hundreds of times over the last few weeks throughout South Africa. When the day is over, the men and women leave wearing their crowns. One young man lays his crown in my hands. "Yes, please," he pleads. "I want you to have it." He explains his drawing of two doves in a tree as the blessing of having two parents, and a small dove is himself. "Yes, please," he says. "I want you to have it." He places the crown in my hand.

Over dinner, Bruce, Anita, and I discuss how we could possibly supply enough Memory Books with the enormous need in The Congo. Inside my breaking heart, that is always the question: *How can we reach every grieving child? How can we help children discover their story is important? They are important to God.*

As the second day of training winds down, a principal requests Joan and me to come to his school. "You must come," he implores. "The children have been working on a school presentation for the past two years to do for the first person that visits our school in Buvunga (Bu-voon-ga)." Anita sees no way to accommodate this request due to the presence of rebel forces to the north. At first it seems impossible; but after discussions, Anita decides we must attempt to visit Buvunga. Joan announces she will "go anywhere with Tamara, knowing she will provide adequate prayer." I smile inside, knowing Joan has questioned the presence of a God who would allow such suffering around the world, including her own devastating losses and suffering.

After a Sunday of church and lunch afterwards at an exclusive restaurant on the water, Anita, Joan, the Paden's driver, and myself leave Monday morning for Buvunga. The eighteen-mile drive north will take four hours due to rough roads. Just outside Goma Anita points out a U.N. outpost housing hundreds of peacekeeping forces. They are in The Congo in an attempt to neutralize the rampages of terror rebels indiscriminately inflict on civilians. Anita tells us the rebels fled from Rwanda where they were involved in the brutal massacre of a million Tutsis in 1994. The U.N. forces have been successful at driving them from areas, but they simply reconstitute themselves somewhere else. Peacekeeping has had little effect on bringing peace back to the citizens of The Congo.

Across the dusty road a tree straddles two makeshift saw horses. Uniformed police officers approach our vehicle. A man peers inside the vehicle as he speaks to Anita in French. Joan and I quietly sit in the back. I am wearing my stethoscope around my neck hoping it sends a message of the nature of our visit. No one can see the anxiety mounting inside when I fear the uniformed man's power to ask us out of the car. Anita and the officer continue to talk. From her purse, Anita retrieves an individual packet of Tylenol and hands it to the man. He motions with an ambivalent wave of his hand that the gate be moved, and turns to walk away. Anita explains he complained of feeling sick. She has learned in her many years living in The Congo that everyone wants something. You simply have to figure out what it is.

As the jeep jumps and lurches all over the road, Anita tells us about the time her daughter and she were stopped at a roadblock and the officers held them for eight hours. Anita decided to appeal to the men by using her knowledge of Congolese culture. She began to wail about not being able to see her son ever again. Over and over again, she cried and made a huge scene. Eventually they let the two of them go because they simply couldn't take her wailing anymore.

A truck piled high with agricultural products and men, women, and children riding on top, barely passes us. Anita tells us about two young girls who had their legs severed while the truck in which they were riding passed too closely to another.

We arrive at another roadblock, but this time the officer asks the driver for registration papers and his license. After he studies them, he and our driver and Anita argue in French. Several other uniformed officers walk around the vehicle. Joan and I remain quiet and appear disinterested. The officer returns the papers and angrily waves the gate to be opened. Anita explains he challenged that the registration was expired and was going to arrest and jail our driver. The driver told him he couldn't jail him because he was from that town and knew that no jail existed. He turns to us in the back seat and laughs.

Soon there appeared to be no one left traveling this road. No trucks or cars. No ox pulled carts or even people walking. Without accompanying conversation, I watch as we pass beautiful dense forests. The forests were once the homes of the gorilla population but rebels have killed them, too, Anita later laments.

The dirt road appears to end, and without warning I realize we have arrived. Several children in the street suspiciously watch as we climb from our vehicle. A group of children appear from a trail and take our hands to lead us. The principal of Buvunga School, who is still wearing his crown, greets us. As we are led up the path through tall banana trees, past small one-room block houses with grass or tin roofs, I see a tall girl ahead carrying a sign atop a wooden stick, and behind her marching several dozen children playing music from handmade kazoos. As we pass by, they turn and lead us through the open schoolyard to wooden chairs in front of the school building. The marching band circles the yard not just blowing their kazoo, but actually playing music together.

I laugh to myself. I have had many introductions, but never a marching band! Lowering their kazoos, the children, all dressed in tattered royal blue and white school uniforms, begin to sing. From a door of the school two lines of young girls join the singing as they move rhythmically into position before us. Gently, the girls brush hands together and slide side-to-side singing the most beautiful song I have ever heard. I study the girl's faces and find most radiantly beaming from somewhere deep within. I completely discard my original thoughts of tattered clothes when I am completely overwhelmed by the moment of beauty offered to us. The young girl directly in front of me lowers her eyes; when our eyes meet. I sense she knows I am watching her. When the song is finished she raises her head and I catch her gaze. I quietly smile a message: I see you, child. God sees you. You are His beautiful creation whom He deeply loves. Here in this place called Buvunga at the end of a dirt road at the end of the world, I whisper, *God knows your name.*

The girls return to the school while the marching band members kneel at the edge of the schoolyard. A group of young boys march the perimeter dressed in green helmets made from woven banana leaves, holding over their shoulders wooden guns carved from banana tree stocks. I see hanging from belts grenades carved from avocadoes. Called to halt by a taller boy wearing wire-rimmed glasses, we watch as the young boys portray inside knowledge of life as a child soldier. Appearing to murder farm workers and kidnap young girls, the boys return them to the wire-rimmed actor playing their superior officer. My heart breaks when I realize each child is telling a story of personal knowledge from his own life.

A boys' choir wrote the music and words to a song describing their life as orphans not as you might think, but grateful for life itself. As they conclude, they begin to dance, stomping and twirling accompanied by a large drum as dust rises above the banana trees. Soon nearly everyone present could no longer stand by without joining the gleeful celebration, including the principal and our own driver stomping and twirling. The young girl who had innocently danced in front of me walks up to me and takes both my hands in hers. Looking up into my eyes, she speaks in French and unknowingly echoes the wise words of South African Archbishop Desmond Tutu. "We must forgive one another," she whispers innocently. She is right. We must forgive those who have wronged us. Without forgiveness there is only a future of bitterness, hatred, and revenge.

Before we leave the school we visit each classroom filled with students. The older students have desks, but younger students simply sit on wooden benches. One young boy shows us a wooden toy truck with much pride. Upon leaving a young girl hands the principal a human skull she just found in the bushes near the schoolyard.

After lunch with the pastor and his family, we reluctantly head for the car so we will be back in Goma before dark. The street children follow us down the trail, and run screaming from Joan as she blows bubbles from a small bottle into the air. As the car begins to move, I turn to wave through the back window. One young girl places her hand on the window in an attempt for our hands to meet. For a moment, only glass separates our hands. She runs behind the car for as long as she can keep up, and then I make the decision to turn away so she wouldn't get hurt.

As we travel down the dirt road toward the threat of roadblocks or rebels, I have no thought for my wellbeing but simply dwell on those who had taught me about courage today. Tears etch a trail through the dust of Buvunga that has gently settled on my face. Joan and I are forever bonded to the children of Buvunga. I will never ever forget the day. I will never ever forget the faces. I will never ever forget their stories.

Before leaving Goma, Anita and I agree The Hope Center will distribute 1,800 Memory Books among the children attending the center. We will continue to explore the opportunity to provide Memory Books to use within the schools, possibly targeting children entering fifth grade. Anita has begun talks with the local pastor to build and operate a Hope Center in Buvunga.

Returning to South Africa, Joan and I conduct training about child grief and loss with twenty house mothers at Lily of the Valley, and dozens of medical, social, psychology professionals sponsored by McCord Hospital and Sinikithemba HIV/AIDS Clinic in Durban. My dream of planting the seed that every grieving child has the potential for healing by telling their story has finally found a place to be nurtured. When grannies caring for children at Lily stand and tell of their own grief from loss of nearly everything dear to them, they understand the importance of the role of simply sitting close to a child while they tell their story. Whether words or drawings, the greatest gift you can give a child is to be a witness to their story, Joan says.

During a quiet early morning before my flight, Malcolm and I discuss the potential, as it seems Memory Books are spreading across the continent of Africa. His words, "Better to spread an inch wide and a mile deep, then a mile wide and an inch deep," encourage me to think of how well we touch children's lives, not how many lives we touch

While aboard a flight to Cape Town, I sit next to a South African woman who fled with her two beautiful daughters when she learned her equestrian groomsman had attempted to brutally murder an elderly neighbor. She fumbles at the buttons on the wrist of her jacket, while she explains the friend and neighbor heard something outside her bedroom window. As she lifted the curtain, someone reached through the burglar bars and pulled her head against the bars, attacking her with a hatchet and nearly killing her. The woman said, "After I had to let the man go because of poor performance, I found a bloody hatchet hidden under his mattress. Although he was convicted and imprisoned, I fear for my life and my daughters and we moved to Cape Town. Unable to sell, I return to check on the house occasionally. I don't know that I'll ever return to live there. Oh, I'm sorry to upset you," she responds to my tears.

"Oh, it's really okay," I reply. "I guess the horror of the story struck a nerve with me. I encountered something while here that really upset me." I begin to tell her about being pulled over by the two men. Between the facts, I attempt to make sense of what didn't make sense. I talked until there wasn't anything else to say.

The woman leans across the empty seat between us and quietly speaks, "Just this last weekend a young girl leaving an equestrian center where she boarded her horse disappeared near the same place you were stopped. She was found in a nearby sugar cane field bound, raped, and murdered." I begin to feel sick to my stomach and momentarily think I might be sick. "Black men want to punish white men by killing the women in their lives," she said looking into my tearing eyes. Placing her hand on my arm, she said, "You, my dear, are the luckiest woman I know. God must have something very important for you to do."

I respond to her, "I don't know that I'm lucky, but I do know God helped me that day."

During previous trips, I immediately flew home to the waiting and needy arms of my family. Most often I immediately returned to responsibilities without so much as a day to debrief and rest. This trip I had planned to stay in Cape Town to rest and recover. I would have no idea how important this particular decision would be. Malcolm suggested I stay at the beautiful Cape Grace Hotel on the waterfront in Cape Town. I order dinner in my room and after a hot bath I slide into the large bed piled with luxurious bedding and attempt a sound sleep. My dreams fill with images of hatchet wielding men, the elderly woman screaming while being bludgeoned. I wake to the sound of my own moans, believing I am being handcuffed. The next morning I sleep late and enjoy breakfast in my room. I walk across a bridge to a waterfront shopping area where I purchase a beautiful tapestry called Mother Africa created by a micro-business of African women. As they hang from scaffolding, the women meticulously thread back and forth, creating absolutely breathtaking tapestries. After lunch I lounge at the poolside and mindlessly look through magazines and nap as I rehearse in my mind the attempt at my abduction. I order dinner in my room and enjoy a beautiful sunset before retiring. I wake to the day I return home to those I love. I am excited to be home, yet I knew I must tell my husband and sons about the danger I encountered on this trip. I know it might change everything.

I no longer return home from these trips to everyone waiting at the airport. Ron greets me at the security area. After a warm bath at home, I climb into bed to recover from the thirty-two hour flight from southern Africa to Oregon. I wonder when I will find the right time to tell him about the day I nearly lost my life. I fear so deeply it will keep me from ever returning to Africa.

Over lunch with Ron at Sunny Hans, my favorite teriyaki chicken restaurant, I now recognize there is no right time for bad news. "Honey, I have something to tell you. You are not going to be happy about it." I could see his expression change. I wonder by his response if he thinks I am going to tell him I had been unfaithful. No, I thought. But I wonder if this news is even more devastating. "While driving to Phinda I was pulled over by rogue policemen and they tried to abduct me." I watch his face sadden. "I was able to talk them into allowing me to pay them off. I'm sorry, honey. I have never wanted to worry you. I don't know if I will ever be able to go back to South Africa again.'"

"I don't know if I can let you," he said.

Somewhere inside I feel I have betrayed his faith in what I believed in. Until now I never felt I was at risk of losing what I loved most—my husband, my family—by following the quiet call to go to the far side of the sea. I grieved knowing I had produced so much pain for my loving, devoted husband. And I know it wouldn't end here, because I have three sons who will also be distressed when I tell them.

The words were not easy, recounting the event that could have changed all of our lives forever. "Mom! I knew something like this was going to happen!" Their responses were all similar. Anger. Fear. Disgust. I realize there is a great sacrifice by those who love me when I choose to follow God's call on my life. Over the years, I experienced the loss of friends, but to lose the faith in you by family is devastating.

I feel personally responsible for what has happened so I never bring it up again. But quietly and painfully I suffer from Post-Traumatic Stress Disorder (PTSD), diagnosed by a psychologist friend. Without warning I experience anxiety attacks, sleeplessness, nightmares, and fear. I fear letting anyone know because I feel they have sacrificed enough. I feel alone, yet I am reminded of how God rescued me on that day. I remind myself of the woman's words, "God must have something very important for you to do. You are the luckiest woman I know." She may think it luck; I know it to be God.

The Democratic Republic of the Congo

Shortly after Joan and I leave Goma and return home, we learn the danger Bruce and Anita live with everyday is real. During the night, they are awakened by a loud crash. Along with their security guard, they find their neighbor has driven his car through the ten-foot tall block wall and into their yard. Upon inspection, they realize he had been shot in the head and killed while driving on the street in front of their home.

As I read the description of events, the remnants of post traumatic stress explode and I immediately begin to rehearse the attempted abduction I encountered. Anxiety and fear cloud my thinking. My heart rate is racing. My legs begin to tremble. And then I remind myself I am not trapped in that situation. I am here. I am home. I am safe.

The fifty boxes containing 1,800 French and Swahili memory books are retrieved a few boxes at a time by Bruce and Anita from Gisneyi across the border from Goma. It is more likely they would arrive undisturbed in Gisneyi, but they still have to get them successfully through customs at the border. Tensions are high from rebel fighting just outside the city of Goma. Bruce and Anita are on high alert for evacuation if the fighting breaches city limits, threatening everyone in Goma. With the last batch of boxes still in the van from the day's trip to Gisneyi, Bruce and Anita receive word the rebels are fighting nearby and they must flee Goma immediately. Bruce and Anita send word they have made it to Kigali and will stay there until the threat subsides. As months go by, the Padens decide to evacuate to the US and visit family in Europe until things calm down. I receive periodic emails describing the fear they have for friends they have left behind in Goma. They have no idea if their home or The Hope Center still exists, and they have difficulty in receiving news about Goma due to poor internet communication usually only available in Gisneyi.

The news from Buvunga, where the marching kazoo band met us, is not good. The rebels have stormed through the tiny village on a murdering rampage. The pastor's survival no less than a miracle when he hides under a bed in his tiny home and escapes certain death when bullets tear through the brick and mortar. All I can think of is the school children, especially the young girl who danced and sung in front of me not so long ago. *Oh, God!* I cry. *I do not want to imagine the horror of such an event. Please, God,* I plead, *save and protect the children of Buvunga. Save and protect the children in the world.*

After months of chaos, Bruce and Anita receive word things have calmed down and they return to Goma. I receive a message from them that when they arrive to a relatively undisturbed home they find the van filled with Memory Books completely untouched in the midst of war and mass destruction. An answer to our prayers!

Chapter 20

Life Sentence for the Innocent

Attending a mission breakfast at church in the fall of 2008, I meet Emmanuel, a Rwandan who survived the 1994 genocide of one million Tutsis in Rwanda. While away attending a university in The Congo, Emmanuel returned home for a visit only to be confronted by something he could not understand. His brother retrieved him from the airport, but admonished him to get right back on a plane for The Congo. Since he feared officials stationed at roadblocks all over Kigali would detain Emmanuel, his brother asked a friend who was a French soldier to transport him back to the airport. Passing by the 25,000-seat athletic arena, he questioned the quiet Frenchman about why people filled the arena. He learned later that the people being detained at the arena were later executed.

At the airport and passing through immigration, Emmanuel was asked to present his identification. In Rwanda, Tutsis and Hutus each carried identification by official order. Unaware of the impending doom for Tutsis, Emmanuel reached into his pocket and pulled an identification card showing he was a university student in the Congo. After he had passed through immigration, he placed his university student ID card back in his shirt pocket right next to this Tutsi ID card that he might have retrieved instead. He did not know then that this simple act saved his life. His siblings were killed. His mother was left for dead. Emmanuel survived one of the world's most heinous crimes against humanity: the massacre of Rwandan men, women and children simply because they were Tutsi.

Emmanuel returned to Rwanda and found no one he once knew. He wondered why God would lead him there. Beside him on the roadside were nine orphaned boys. Before night fell he had found shelter among widows for each of the boys, and had promised the women he would help them if the women simply cared for the boys.

Following the breakfast, I have an opportunity to share with Emmanuel about the Memory Book project, and openly wonder why Rwandan children shouldn't have a Memory Book. While traveling through Rwanda last year with Bruce and Anita, I visited the Kigali Parents School, a private school where we eventually placed 300 Memory Books. Emmanuel tells me there is great need in Rwanda to help children suffering from loss of their families. "You will see," he says. Ron and I agree to travel to Rwanda with Emmanuel in June.

After hearing a guest speaker at church, I wait in a long line to ask a pastor from Nigeria if Memory Books would be helpful for children living in his community. While the purpose of his trip has to do with tractors for Nigerian farmers, he agrees to discuss the idea through email. Immediately upon returning to his homeland, I receive a request from him to send as many Memory Books as we can. There is a great need in Nigeria, he says.

In Nigeria, news reports Islamic militants have recently burned churches and killed Christians. He hopes Memory Books will help children who have witnessed such traumatic crises to heal from these devastating events.

During January, Ron and I load his cutting horses into the horse trailer and head to Buckeye, Arizona, so he can ride during the coldest of months in Oregon. Cutting horse trainer Bobby Usher and his wife Kathy offer to let us park in their driveway with other cutting horse enthusiasts. While he rides, I sit outside the trailer in the shade and write a rough draft for a lesson planner based on Malcolm's statement of "one inch wide and a mile deep." While the Memory Book provides children an opportunity to preserve memories of what they have lost, a Memory Book Club continues to invest in the lives of the children as they grow and develop, helping them re-establish a new sense of identity. The two years worth of lessons will be related to topics like identity, self-esteem, confidence, and purpose and will include a craft the children can create to help them remember the lesson. I believe this will promote the "inch wide, mile deep" concept.

When Monday Night's begin again in early spring, the women are surprised to learn they will be building craft kits designed for each lesson. Titles include *Bloom Where You Are Planted* that uses coffee filters edged with water colors and pinched in the center with a wire chenille wrap to make a flower, and *Remembering* that allows a child to make a yellow paper heart shape placed on a yarn hanger to wear or hang in a tree for remembering the person they loved and lost. We begin by making enough for 4,000 children attending current Memory Book Clubs in Nigeria, Tanzania, and South Africa. Requests for additional Memory Books continued to come in so many of the women are happy to continue to do what requires little concentration while they visit with one another.

In June, Ron and I fly to Kigali, Rwanda, with Emmanuel and a few others interested in helping Rwandans reconstruct their lives following the devastating genocide of one million people. There is no amount of preparation you can undergo to ready yourself for what we would encounter. The agenda for the first few days is designed to shed light on the history of the battle by other nations' attempts to colonize this land. By the end of the two weeks, there is no doubt in my mind the entire country of Rwanda is grieving.

Home to two dominant tribes, the Hutus and the Tutsis, the Belgian colonization of Rwanda attempted to bring equality to the smaller tribe of Tutsis by elevating its members to higher standard of living jobs and positions in government. Well-meaning yet terribly misguided, Belgian scientists even deemed the Tutsis of greater intellect due to the size of their brains. All of this lead to enormous resentment by the Hutu tribe so when foreign influence eventually left Rwanda in 1994, the pent up rage exploded and led to the mass murder of one million men, women, and children in 100 days. Tutsis and everyone associated through marriage, business, or sympathetic to Tutsis were brutally and savagely murdered.

Just a few miles from downtown Kigali, we drive through a peaceful rural community dotted with block homes and farmlands. The caravan of cars turns down a gravel road where children dressed in school uniforms walk home from school. The cars stop in front of a brick church building surrounded with green lawn, and purple and white banners waving in a warm gentle breeze. This is a genocide memorial site, Emmanuel announces.

Near to the doorway is a small table with a guestbook opened to today's date. The mood is solemn as we each sign our names. Emmanuel points to the cement walkway littered with hundreds of pockmarks created by machine gun blasts. The iron gate is contorted and broken. As I step into the large sanctuary I am confronted with the reality of what this place memorializes. Lying on top of several dozen pews is the blood stained clothing of 10,000 men, women, and children who died in this place. The washed, but red, rust, brown colored shirts, pants, dresses, vests, purses, children's Sunday best, and baby layettes is three to four feet deep, and thousands of shoes are neatly placed beneath.

My breath is taken away. Somewhere deep inside of me I feel an enormous welling up of grief that somehow cannot escape. My eyes skim the room filled with ribbons of sunlight streaming through the thousand bullet holes penetrating the metal roof.

In a flash, I feel as though I can see the fire of bullets hailing down and marked by the sunlight. I hear the thousands of people who have hidden here in the sanctuary of this small church begin to scream and cry, realizing they are trapped. They were told they would be safe, only to discover they had been lured here to be murdered. From the rooftop, from the windows, and through the walls of bricks, assailants with hatred in their hearts riddle human flesh with bullets, butcher with hatchets and knives until every single man, woman, and child is dead.

I cannot breathe. I flee into the yard where the warm breeze meets the tears falling down my cheeks. I try to replace the thoughts, but suddenly all I can think about is the terror, the screaming, the deep sadness this place is. *Oh, God,* I cry out. *How must this grieve you, my God,* I languish. I wish I could flee, but realize the images of terror are within me. There is nowhere I can go to escape. I realize these images hold hostage the minds of those who have survived—a life sentence for even the innocent.

One by one, others leave the sanctuary, and outside we are led down stairs into a common burial site where all 10,000 skeletons are set upon shelves. I did not know if I wanted to see this sight. Yet, I felt it important to expose myself to the gruesome images, knowing Rwandan children had no choice but to live with such horrific memories.

Outside I see a woman washing the decorative tiles of the large cement lid of the burial site. Emmanuel introduces her as a survivor of the genocide. She lifts her hat to reveal a deep red scar penetrating her skull. The woman tells Emmanuel she still fears she will be killed one day. As we drive away from the church with banners imploring to never forget, Emmanuel expresses his fear that Rwanda is just one bad leader away from another massacre.

On Monday morning, Ron and I travel to a small community outside Kigali where Emmanuel has built a sewing center and woodworking shop for orphaned teens to learn skills. I am immediately led into the classroom where fifteen young girls are learning to sew garments they can sell. Without preparation, I simply began to tell my own childhood story of loss and grief due to divorce and poverty. When I finish I ask if there are any girls with similar stories they would like to tell.

Although hesitant at first, one by one each girl stands and tells a story of terror, poverty, abuse, and hopelessness. All of them were young girls when the genocide occurred, but remember in graphic detail the memories of things they witnessed. My heart grieves knowing those images will never be forgotten. As I hug each girl, I wonder to myself how long it had been since they felt loved. Having brought just a few dozen Memory Books, I offer each of the girls from the sewing class a Memory Book of their own. One girl who had not shared her story told the interpreter she wanted to share her story. She stood and told her story as tears streamed down her face. When she finished I hugged her, too, while she hid her face against my chest and sobbed. Then without warning, she pulled away from me and steadied herself brushing away her tears, and returned to her seat. Her moment to grieve was over.

Ron tells everyone his only purpose for coming to Rwanda is for my safety. While I am in the sewing center, Ron is being fully drafted to help oversee the construction of a woodworking center. Currently, the woodworking center for the dozen boys is open air under a tarp, with handmade manual tools. With forty years of experience in commercial construction, Emmanuel couldn't have anyone better than Ron suited for the job. And frankly, I am pleased when Ron discovers God has another reason for him coming to Rwanda.

When we arrive at the site the next day to receive a bulldozer to clear and flatten the land, Ron finds thirty barefoot men leveling the land with hoes and shovels. When he borrows survey equipment, he has to convince the foreman of the jobsite the plot lines are accurate. The cement is hand mixed and carried in buckets and shallow bowls by barefoot men and women to pour over rocks, creating the foundation. The stem wall pillars are individually handmade from wire and rebar using primitive tools. Thousands of bricks are made from dirt and water poured into molds then left in the hot sun to dry for three days before being used to construct the walls. Designs are drawn for roofing, electricity, and overhead doors to be completed later. During a late afternoon meeting, I remember Bruce and Anita are closing a similar woodworking shop due to violence in Goma, and wonder if their machinery might be available. Emmanuel emails them and amazingly their machinery is available, if funding and bringing it across the border to Kigali is possible.

One afternoon, I am invited to a church to meet 250 children whom Emmanuel thought might benefit by having a Memory Book. I load some art supplies and craft kits containing crowns into a small bag and leave with an interpreter. When we arrive, I walk along the sidewalk running the length of the church and look into the windows of the church where I see no less than 500 children. Leaving the suitcase with supplies at the door, I enter without the slightest idea what I will do.

The church pastor introduces me and I still don't know what I'm going to do! Without a plan, I begin to sing, *I Am Somebody* at the top of my lungs. The words simply dissipate into the booming noise of children. The interpreter shouts, "I am somebody" in Kenyarwanda, Rwanda's official language, and the children begin to quiet. "I am somebody," I shout, "and I know that my worth is not found on this earth, I'm a child of the Most High God."

I shout, "You are somebody!" I point to a child, then another, and another. "You are somebody. And you know that your worth is not found on this earth, you are a child of the Most High God." The children are all erupting in laughter. Startled when I point to each child, some of the older boys sit with arms crossed, suspicious of this white woman. "I am somebody," I begin to teach the children in English. Broken yet recognizable, they begin to repeat in English the words to the theme song we adopted for Memory Book Club. The room erupts into chaos. The interpreter calls the children to order and tells them I have come with a message. I have? I muse. Quickly, I think to myself: *if I were to never ever see these children again, what do I have to give them? What would I tell them?*

"When I was nine years old," I begin, "my father and mother divorced. My mother worked long days and my siblings and I had to take care of each other. I felt alone and wondered if anyone loved me. In my neighborhood, there was a grannie who had a Bible club after school at her house. She invited me to write a Scripture on a card and memorize it. If I could say it to her, then she gave us milk and cookies. I don't remember her name, but I do remember she made me feel like I was somebody. Not just a nobody, but a special somebody who was loved by God. Today, I want to tell you, you are somebody. Not just a nobody, but a very special somebody, whom God loves. I don't care if you remember my name, but I want you to remember this. Remember the day a lady came and told you how much God loves you, and that you are his child."

I turn to the interpreter as if to say, okay, is that it? He responds, "You can have them all afternoon." Okay, I'm thinking. What else? "Can I pray for them?" I ask the interpreter?

"Yes. Yes," he responds happily.

"Who needs prayer because they are sick?" I ask. A long line forms and I place my hands on their heads or their shoulders and begin to pray over each child. "Who needs prayer because they are lonely?" Again, a long line forms and I pray over each child. "Who needs prayer for sadness? Who needs prayer for school studies? Who needs prayer for their families?" The lines grow longer and longer, yet I pray for every single child. From the back of the room, two women carry a child forward and lay him on the floor in front of me. He is disabled with cerebral palsy. He was abandoned. He had asked the women to carry him forward for prayer. I kneel before this young boy and begin to pray. His body shakes violently as I pray. The otherwise noisy room has quieted and everyone's eyes are on the young boy. The interpreter and women help him to his feet and help him back to his seat.

I announce, "We should thank God for the answers to our prayers, whether today or tomorrow or in his perfect time. Lets dance and celebrate." I began to shout and dance and within seconds I am surrounded by hundreds of dancing, shouting children. Whether their day started out feeling like celebrating, it will end celebrating together. Thank you, God, I whisper. As we leave, the interpreter comments it was very good for the children, very good.

Before we leave Rwanda, I meet 450 children who were either placed with widows or are waiting to be placed in Emmanuel's organization, and arrange for shipment of 1,500 Memory Books, including art supplies, for these Rwandan children and others.

Nigeria

The first shipment of Memory Books to Nigeria is sent directly into a hotbed of radical-Islamic terrorism against Christians in the mountainous northern region. The pastor in Nigeria emails me to report 3000 Memory Books have arrived. His wife invites and prepares to train church leaders to distribute and use Memory Books among many church youth programs within the region. They email photos taken during training sessions with Memory Books stacked before participants. Some photos show the adults enjoying the crown kits made for every child receiving a personal Memory Book.

Within weeks we are receiving thank you letters handwritten by children expressing their gratitude for a Memory Book. A young girl is amazed to learn God knows what is in her heart, her hopes, and dreams. One teenage girl reports she was once going against her parents, lying to them. She says that when she received her Memory Book something changed in her. "It happened so fast I do not know what it was, but I no longer want to go against my parents," she writes. Many of the letters reveal a deep desire to leave Nigeria and come to America, or request items that will help their lives. One small group of children touch our hearts in particular because of the simplicity of their requests: size seven shoes, pencils, a Bible, or children's books. The Monday Night group purchases all the items mentioned and a few extra things for children who did not write. We include a Max Lucado book we believe the adults will enjoy. It would be so easy to forget such simple requests, especially at a time holiday busyness distracts us. I am reminded of my need for decent shoes as a child, and realize a young boy's prayer for new shoes would be an amazing prayer to answer. I try to imagine the moment he will open the box containing the checkered black and white canvas slip-ons. Not only new, but quite cool. I can picture him growing in self-esteem with each step.

Chapter 21

Talking Stick

It is the summer of 2010 and I have agreed to return to Rwanda without Ron to conduct training seminars in child grief and loss to church leaders who work with children. Over the past year, I have continued to develop a training method that will help adults understand the role they play in helping a child process their grief, and the use of a Memory Book as a tool for the grief journey.

During the next two weeks, Emmanuel has arranged for two-day training sessions in three different churches with people who work in children's programs. While the focus of the efforts over the years has been in orphanages, the reality is every child is grieving loss in Rwanda and many other countries around the world.

Inside a large church, a small group of men and women sit with pencils posed ready to take notes. With Clement as my interpreter, I begin to describe the difference between mourning and grieving, and why a smiling child may indeed be grieving deeply inside. I explain while the external response of mourning may look different among cultures, and influenced by traditions and mores, the act of grieving is an innate universal human internal response to loss that does not differ whether we are Rwandan or American. I explain grieving is like atmospheric pressure. You can't see or touch either one, but their presence produces havoc. The greater the change in atmospheric pressure the greater the damaging results. The greater the loss the greater the grief, and the greater potential for life altering symptoms like sleeplessness, stomach ailments, fatigue, lack of concentration, depression, headaches, and anger. All these symptoms, and many more, are often not associated with grieving, so the source of those ailments—grief—is not acknowledged and may lie hidden deep inside for a lifetime.

After a morning tea break, while holding a brightly painted "talking stick" I explain the use of the talking stick with children. The talking stick originated with American Indians who used it in their council meetings. The one holding the talking stick is given the right and honor to speak without fear of interruption, judgment or ridicule while others listen. And anyone who talks holds the responsibility of speaking truth.

"When I was nine years old," I begin, "my father and mother divorced. My father married another woman and started a new family…." I tell the story of my childhood. When I finish I ask if there is anyone with a similar story. Quietly, patiently I wait, looking about the room as most look down to their papers. Then a young man slowly raises his hand, "Yes, I have a story," he said as he stands. I hand him the talking stick, and he begins to tell the story of his father leaving when he was seven years old. His mother could not feed all of his brothers and sisters, so she gave him to a farmer who took him into a field to watch his goats and left him there for two years. He slept under a tree with the goats. He was covered with sores and bugs. His clothes were torn and dirty. He starved.

As he speaks, I stand with my arms folded behind my back exhibiting body language of openness and fully attentive. When his face expresses sadness, I mirror that emotion back to him. I neither look at my watch, or fidget with my clothing, or look about impatiently as he takes as long as the story needs. When he is done, I simply extend a lingering handshake, look into his eyes, and say, "Thank you for telling us your life story."

"Anyone else?" I ask. "Would anyone else like to tell his or her story?" The room is quiet. A young man stands and begins to tell how he had survived the genocide even though he had been beat with a hatchet and left for dead in a pit of bloody bodies. For years his sleep is interrupted by the nightmares of gruesome contorted faces frozen from a horrific death. A woman tells us the story of being left by her husband to care for their children alone, unable to remarry because of the culture. One by one, each stands and tells a story of survival, of brutality, of despair, of loss, of grief. Each and every time I fold my arms behind my back to convey I am open to the person and hearing the tragic and often gruesome details each shares.

"The greatest gift you can give a child," I said, "is to sit close and be a witness to their story."

A middle-aged man sitting in the back asks, "Doesn't the retelling of such difficult stories just do more trauma to a child?"

"That is a very good question," I reply. "Tell me, sir. When you stood and told your story while everyone listened, how did it make you feel?"

"I felt better," he said, nodding his head.

"Yes. You feel better. And so will the children."

Emmanuel arranges for a lovely meal of roasted chicken, rice, vegetables, and fruit to be served. Grief work is hard work, so after listening and telling personal life stories everyone is famished. I take a small serving, but spend most of the time watching as everyone laughs and talks with a sense of relief as they realize they are not alone in their losses. There is someone who has suffered a similar fate. They no longer had to endure the gruesome details of their story alone. Those details have been exposed, and no one refused to neither acknowledge their existence no matter how horrific nor reject a willingness to share the burden of the reality.

While everyone escapes for a few moments outdoors, a middle-aged man comes to me and quietly asks if he can speak. "I am a husband who has left a wife with daughter," he begins. "I married another woman and I now live on the other side of the city. I do not have the means to visit my daughter. When I try to see her, she won't talk. She is angry with me. She does not understand I cannot visit frequently."

"When did you last see your daughter?" I ask.

"A year ago," he responds. As he spoke I deemed he was attempting to gain sympathy for his plight, yet I immediately related to his daughter's heartbreak.

"I have an answer for you," I told him. "You may not like what I have to say. You have broken your daughter's heart. By your actions you have told her without words, 'You are not important to me.' I am your daughter, sir, when she grows up. She will be wounded by your lack of love and attention."

"But," he interrupts, "I have no way to see her often. I have no car or money for a taxi."

"Do you have a bike?"

"No," he laughs.

"Can you afford a stamp?" I ask.

"Yes, I can afford a stamp."

"Then write to your daughter. Write to her every week. Ask her to forgive you. Tell her how sorry you are that your choices have hurt her so deeply. Tell her how much you love her. Make a plan to save enough money to visit when you can. There is no excuse for not pursuing a relationship with your daughter. It simply needs to be a priority."

"You are right," he responds.

"Trust me when I say being a father to your daughter is the single most important thing you will ever do with your life," I say.

After lunch, Clement helps me hand out blank paper and colored pencils. I suggest that some stories are too difficult to talk about. Young children may lack the verbal or language skills to accurately tell their story. I suggest children might want to tell a story in a drawing, a story that needs no words. I give each in attendance an opportunity to draw a picture. When they finish, I ask again, "Is there anyone who would like to share their picture?" One by one, each stands to share what they had drawn. A young man had drawn a picture of his dismembered father with three men running away. The knives they welded had red blood dripping from the tips.

"This is my father," he said as his eyes went from the graphic drawing to my eyes and back again. My eyes steady on the drawing and then to his eyes. It was as though he was asking, "Are you willing to share this horrific story of my life with me?" He continues in a quiet, quivering voice, "These men killed my father, my mother, and my sisters; I hid under the bed. I have always felt guilty. Had I not hid under my bed I might have been able to save my father."

"How old were you?" I ask.

"I was four."

"You were four," I respond. "You must have been very afraid, as a four year old."

"Yes, I was very afraid," he said.

"Do you think as a four year old you could have saved your father from those men?" I ask, waiting patiently for him to rationalize an answer.

"No, " he shook his head. I watched as tears welled up in his eyes.

Quietly, I simply let his answer linger in the air. "Thank you," I said, "for sharing the story of your family and what happened to them. I can see your story makes you feel very sad." He simply shook his head yes.

Outside the room, no one can ignore the cries of a small child. Clement and I find a boy and girl behind the building. She explains amidst the sobbing of the boy that someone stole his pencil. I immediately retrieve from my supplies a newly sharpened pencil and hand it to him. His is the face of grief. Not over his lost pencil, but when even small losses occur the sadness goes down inside and hooks into a massive presence of grief from a tremendous loss, and an unexpected response occurs. This child grieved deeply even though it was just a pencil. Grief is not compartmentalized but is stored as a whole.

A young girl, who had yet to speak at all, raises her hand. "This is my life," she says as she points to a basket. "All these things surrounding the basket are things I wish for my life." She points to flowers, a red heart, and other things she has drawn.

"You have many dreams for your life," I said.

"Yes, but I am sad because the basket is empty. I have no family. I go home after school with friends and hope they will invite me to eat dinner. Often times I will ask if I can stay the night. I have no home of my own." She sits down, covers her face with her hands, and begins to sob openly. I kneel in front of her and try to offer comfort. She cries and cries in her hands. A woman in the back of the room stands and suggests we pray for her. The woman comes forward and says she had been without food for some time and had prayed for God to give her food. When we served the meal today, she said she cried because God had answered her prayer. The woman prays that God would fill the young girl's basket to overflowing. As I leave the building for the day, the young girl and her two friends stay behind to talk. She thanks me for giving her the opportunity to tell her story. Then the three of them link arm-in-arm and walk away.

During the second day, I introduce the Memory Book and its use for children to write or draw their stories. It provides children an opportunity to preserve memories of their childhood that otherwise may be lost. Preserving those memories allows children to see they were mere children when traumatic events or crises occurred, and that their perspective may contain untruths or limited understanding because of their age. If the memories are preserved, children can revisit those memories and gain greater understanding and truth about what happened to them as they grow and mature.

Along with the Memory Book, adults working with children are encouraged to learn about and offer a Memory Book Club for children which provides children an opportunity to tell their story during talking stick time, make crafts, and hear lessons related to their identity, purpose, and hope for a future. For the next hour, I introduce a Memory Book Club setting for the adults. We sing *I Am Somebody*, make coffee filter flowers, and paper plate crowns—all with much laughter and fun. I share the lesson titled *Bloom Where You Are Planted*, telling them the story about an alpine flower living at the rocky and often stormy high elevation on Kilimanjaro, just where God planted it to live and fulfill its purpose. I tell them each of us are given life, often in a stormy and inhospitable environment. Yet, God created us to fulfill a purpose for our lives in that place. Bloom where you are planted, I suggest, can encourage children to not simply hope they can move to America, but find purpose in the country in which they live. And just as the alpine flower finds refuge in a crevasse near a rock, lean into God. He can be our Rock.

After the training sessions, Gaspard, a friend of Emmanuel, agrees to help facilitate distribution of Memory Books among the churches represented by the men and women attending the training. Gaspard invites me to speak on his radio program that evening, reaching thousands of Rwandans. When I leave Rwanda, I am burdened by how we can reach all the grieving children left behind by the genocide of those they loved.

Rwanda

Although Emmanuel's organization in Rwanda has a large truck, it is leased to someone so retrieving fifty boxes of Memory Books from the post office has created a dilemma. It is necessary to rent a vehicle to transport the boxes to the headquarters, which proves to be quite costly for the small organization. Gaspard will attempt to distribute them, although I know he is without a vehicle, too. It appears the last mile of the Memory Books' worldwide journey may prove to be the most difficult to accomplish.

This delivery challenge highlights the need for other methods in addition to Memory Books for helping children tell their stories in the midst of loss. There are places in the world where simply handing a child a talking stick may give them everything they need to tell their story. Many cultures around the world use verbal transfer of stories as a means of sharing family history. Even in those cultures, the use of drawings by young children who lack verbal and language skills to communicate may be helpful, as it was for many Rwandans who attended the training.

Chapter 22

Stories Among Us

The house is filled with activity. The entry tables are home to counting popsicle sticks into bags of 600 needed for a craft titled "Guard Your Heart" that encourages children to protect what they put in their minds by building a fence of good judgment. Painted talking sticks are being designed by layering painted strips, polka-dots, even paw prints, making each as unique as the women painting them. A table in the living room allows women to take a moment to write a response to hundreds of letters received from children living in the refugee camp in Tanzania.

Everyone is busy, yet our thoughts are of one of the women whose own daughter has died unexpectedly. One of the women leaves what she is doing and goes to get our grieving friend. As she walks through the door, everyone has stopped what they are doing and surrounds her, each taking turns to embrace our friend. Without doubt, an evening of sharing life and loss with a friend eclipses the need to count or paint wood. Yet, we are discovering when we come together to create these beautiful gifts for grieving children around the world, God does not overlook our own grief and loss. In the midst of this work, God is truly touching our lives when our own childhood grief and loss is uncovered, and when life deals a painful blow. As our friend speaks of her loss, she admits comfort knowing her daughter is with the angels now. Just then a feather floats freely down from somewhere in the room, and she catches it in her hand. She's with Jesus and the angels.

When a church mission team comes to assemble one hundred Memory Books for Esperanza Viva Children's Home in Mexico, Terri accompanies her daughter Rose. Expecting a "scrapbook cult," she is shocked when she finds the effort to provide Memory Books to grieving children around the world a truly rewarding escape from her own troubles. Rose designs a necklace craft for the Spanish language Memory Books and invites other high school teens to help assemble the kits as a part of leadership requirements for high school graduation. Kelsey, Stacy's daughter fluent in French, offers to translate the Training Manual into French for her senior graduation project. Celena, a young teen girl, invites friends to come share the experience of putting together Memory Books or crafts. At times, the house is filled on Monday Night with the vitality of young girls sitting among widows, mothers, and an occasional husband gleaning and giving advice. Occasionally, someone will say something that prompts the singing of a song. Jokes are made about newcomers being scared away by our craziness or my drum, but often followed up with "newbies" returning time and time again.

With no sign up, there is no way of knowing who or how many will come each Monday Night. We've simply learned to trust that who comes and what is done is up to God. At the end of another year, over 7,500 Memory Books are shipped to Nigeria, The Congo, and Rwanda with additional requests from Tanzania, South Africa. During the year-end celebration, I announce a request to come to India in 2011.

A Gift from Tanzania

As I open the large box, a faint odor of incense escapes. The letter on Group Misa stationary is addressed to me. "Dearest Tamara, On behalf of all of us at Group Misa I extend with deepest sadness our condolences for the loss of your mother and our dearest friend Jean." Draped in a purple cloth, I lift up an absolutely beautifully handmade carved wooden set of fruits, vegetables, fish, tray, a pot of flowers with a small, carved bird, and a lovely carved white dove. Pastor Iongwa said the gift was an offering on behalf of my mother, representing how we would enjoy a meal, flowers, and hope between Group Misa residents and my family. I am forever thankful for my Congolese friends living with their own loss and grief living away from their beloved homeland, The Congo, who sent such a beautiful and sacrificial gift honoring my mother, who wrote hundreds of letters to children who call Group Misa home.

Chapter 23

A Fine Line

Once again I have the opportunity to not travel alone, but join a group traveling to India. My husband and family would prefer I wouldn't go at all, but know that simply isn't an option for me. Years ago I asked if this work continues to be God's, it would come to me. Even my husband cannot deny this must be God.

During my trip to Rwanda, I met TJ Saling Caldwell who was asked to interview and photograph all 450 of the orphaned children in Emmanuel's outreach to help facilitate finding the children sponsors. When her church began organizing a trip to India, TJ agreed to return for a second trip to India to interview and photograph children living at two orphanages. She discussed the Memory Book project with leaders and invited me to a planning meeting. Attending the meeting was Dr. Kaye Wilson Anderson who was leading a team of eight nursing students from University of Portland, where she is a professor. I graduated from University of Portland Nursing School, I tell her. "No way!" she said with her Mississippi accent. After describing the Memory Book project, the entire team agrees India children need Memory Books.

The world is certainly no less dangerous at this time, yet I feel a strong calling to go to India. In the midst of hotel bombings in Mumbai and other terror events around the world, I feel I must respond to this request. I have no fear of flying, but the thought of an eight-hour bus ride through rural India gives me reason to feel insecure. I simply pray to God to protect me.

There is nothing that feels good after flying halfway around the world through layovers and plane changes. Inside the bus with curtains drawn,

I feel as though I am riding a theme park ride simulating a journey over mountainous terrain, with sharp jerks and braking in an attempt to keep us from careening over a cliff. I am thankful I cannot actually see the road or terrain because it is pitch black on the trip from Hyderabad south to Narasaropet. After a rose petal greeting by children from a large orphanage, my roommate Ruth and I crash in our room while the nursing students and Dr. Kaye set up the clinic site at orphanage to be ready to see patients the next day. Ruth is experiencing her first international trip as a recent widow, hoping to find the courage to face life alone. After a bath using a five-gallon bucket and cup, we lay on our beds listening to a pigeon coo inside the air-conditioner that is quiet due to a blackout of electricity. In the dark, Ruth tells me about losing the love of her life; I share with her about the devastating and unexpected death of my elder sister Denyce following the loss of our mother. We are both silent in the dark. I can only imagine her face is wet from tears like mine.

Prior to dawn, I wake still exhausted but unable to sleep due to the time zone change. Outside, the wail of a newborn baby from a neighboring building interrupts the silence, then silence. I doze until the sound of a single call to prayer at a local mosque wakes me. I think to myself, if Islam calls its followers to prayer why shouldn't Christianity do the same? I quietly step into the hallway overlooking three floors of rooms. Standing at the balcony, I began to sing.

> Alleluia, alleluia
> For the Lord God Almighty reigns
> Alleluia, Alleluia
> For the Lord God Almighty reigns
>
> Alleluia, holy, holy
> Are You Lord God Almighty.
> Worthy is the Lamb, worthy is the Lamb
> You are holy, holy
> Are You Lord God Almighty.
> Worthy is the Lamb, worthy is the Lamb. Amen.[14]

When I open my eyes, I see several of our team standing in their nightgowns at the handrail of each floor's balcony. My song brought them from their rooms, as well as several Indian men. I close my room door behind me, satisfied I had welcomed the day with prayer to my Lord and Savior, a ritual I repeat with each new morning while in India.

When I arrive at the orphanage, it becomes apparent that plans for the purpose of my coming have been lost in translation. I had planned to conduct a training seminar for adults similar to the one I offered in Rwanda, but quickly change course when I enter a room of 200 children. I am learning to be prepared for anything at any time. While Ruth and a nursing student help the children make bracelets, another nursing student, Twania, and I have a driver literally race back to the hotel, passing on dangerous curves, staring down on coming vehicles and motorcycles to retrieve all the art supplies and craft kits I had brought. Over the next three days, I invite children to tell their story using the talking stick, draw their story, and squeeze in an adult training session related to mourning and grief and the use of the Memory Book. On the last day, Ruth takes photographs of all 200 children and we are able to offer a Memory Book for every child.

After a busy day of seeing hundreds of women who traveled to this site outside Narasaropet for a women's conference and a free health clinic, or working with the Memory Book project, everyone enjoys an evening shopping, ordering custom made saris, facials, and henna paintings.

I am invited to join TJ and others staying at a small informal orphanage four hours from Narasaraopet. Ruth and two nursing students will come for the overnight stay. I will lead child grief and loss training in the rural community. When we arrive, singing children led by the eighty-four-year-old mother of the pastor greet us. We are told she is an orphan and has taught the children over 400 songs. Ruth invites the children to make bracelets. Across the street, a fire is burning rubbish emitting toxic pollutants into the air. It is not until I begin to cough that I notice many of the children are coughing. In the small home, we are given the main bedroom to share, while the nursing students sleep in the adult children's room. There is limited water, so we go to bed without bathing after a one hundred degree day. The grandmother sleeps with the three-dozen children downstairs in rows of bunk beds.

Inside the block building, it is cool yet dark. The training is at a new plot of land just a few minutes away the pastor was given as a donation.

A lone block building attached by a chicken coup sits empty except for roosting pigeons. The pastor's son has agreed to translate into Telegu, the local dialect spoken here, for the eight young people attending the training. Just as I did in Rwanda, I begin by describing the difference between mourning and grief while holding a talking stick. After I tell my own childhood story, I invite others to tell their story. A young man in the front row stands and tells about the death of his father in an auto accident. The room is silent. As he speaks, I battle to stay focused on his story, as my mind goes to the dangerous driving patterns I have observed during my short time in India. I come back to the speaker and hear him say it has been so difficult for his family—to be without his father because he was the one who provided for them. Tears fill his eyes, and he embarrassingly wipes them aside. Immediately, another hand is raised and another story offered—another auto accident. The talking stick is passed about the room, one by one everyone attending the training tells their story of loss. Each story recounts the devastating effects on the person. A young girl stands to tell her story with a faint voice. I expect it may be the first time she has ever spoken the words that have caused so much pain; she gulps for air before the word "died" surfaces.

After lunch, paper and colored pencils are handed out and everyone draws a picture that tells a story. It seems the exercise is fun for the near-adults, as childhood has been absent for some time for these young people. With the training complete, I hand out Certificates of Completion and a Memory Book white hankie monogrammed with "hope" in Telegu to everyone in attendance.

When we return to the house that evening, a turkey that had been wandering around in the courtyard that morning quite alive is served for dinner. TJ warned us to not dream of anything out loud, such as a good old-fashioned American meal, otherwise our hosts would do everything to make it come true. Even at great expense. Sorry, Mr. Turkey.

Calling the children forward to receive their own personal Memory Book is so memorable. I feel honored to be the one to hand this gift made just for them, in the color of their choice. Ruth takes each child's photograph. We invite the children to draw a picture to place in their Memory Book and offer to leave the art supplies. As we gather our things to leave for another orphanage, I watch the children standing on the stairway into the home openly sob when the team that had been there several days hugs each one. As we drive away, I quietly grieve for the children's losses.

We have to be careful we do not grow so close as to create another loss in the lives of these children when we leave. It is a fine line between leaving a child a piece of ourselves instead of affirming God's love for them. God will never leave them. That's what I love about the Memory Book. Its message is about God's enduring love, and unfolds over a lifetime. Those of us involved in Memory Books are simply the messengers.

After an hour's drive back toward Narasaropet, we turn down a dirt road leading to a small home where another pastor and his wife are raising fifteen orphaned children in addition to their own children. We are served lunch of brown rice, steamed shrimp, cooked vegetables, and fruit, but I am suffering from diarrhea and eat nothing. The pastor's daughter leads me by the hand with the others to a large tent set up in a field where I will offer training in child grief and loss in blistering one-hundred degree temperatures. She introduces a gentleman who will translate into Telegu. With most chairs filled, I begin to introduce the difference between mourning and grieving as people continue to come. By the time I tell my own personal childhood experience of loss and grief, the tent is overflowing with one hundred people, many who simply saw something happening and came to see what it was.

For several hours, men and women of all ages stand, hold the talking stick, and tell their own unique story of loss. At one moment the translator anxiously asks, "We came to hear you speak, yes?" With everyone's complete undivided attention, each one shares a story that leaves others shaking their heads in disbelief; those listening often respond with affirmation by clapping. All the while, I am getting sicker and sicker with diarrhea and heat exhaustion. Even water makes a quick exit, yet I continue to pass the talking stick and in the end offer individual prayer for a throng of people pressing all around me.

That evening we are overnight guests of a local Hindu man and his family because the pastor has no room for guests in his small home that already sleeps twenty on the floor. We are told the Hindu man risks retribution for aligning himself with Christians. This sheds light on the threat it is to be a follower of Christ in this land. It is the reason this pastor and his wife take in orphaned children of Christians; their very lives are at risk of slavery or death.

Completely dehydrated and nearly delirious, I lay on a bed shared with Ruth and dream of radical terrorists storming the tent and killing everyone as they profess a faith in Jesus. In darkness, Suzie, a nursing student, wakes me from my moaning and the "too real" dream of horror as my heart pounds inside my chest.

It is Sunday morning, the pastor's wife has handmade each of us a beautiful sari to wear to their church service. Standing with my arms raised, she wraps me in mounds of fabric while singing a beautiful, yet unintelligible, song. I have eaten nothing for two days, yet she struggles to fit all of me into this precious gift from someone who has very little material wealth. I am overcome with that realization as we walk to church along the dirt road holding the hands of orphaned children. Who is the richest in God's kingdom? I remind myself.

With all three hundred Memory Books placed in the hands of grieving Indian children, I am ready to return home. It will take several weeks to return to physical health, and even longer to recover emotionally. The threat to my wellbeing remains only in my dreams. It is a strange feeling to come home to safety and security knowing that throughout the world children of all ages are left alone by death, war, poverty, neglect, or slavery, and that many live at risk every single day, especially as Christians. Several years ago, I lost two friends to breast cancer. I consider the life I live is on borrowed time because of their shortened lives. Why would I ever want to take for granted the years my friends were not given the opportunity to live? Yes, the world is a dangerous place, but if children can trust God to rescue, protect, and care for them, why shouldn't I?

Chapter 24

When Stories Merge

As December approaches, boxes fill with craft kits and art supplies supporting the recently completed Lesson Planner for Memory Book Clubs. Other boxes fill with 1,800 Memory Books. The boxes litter the entire house. All are destined to minister emotional health and hope to grieving children literally all over the world. After returning home from India, we receive additional requests of Memory Books by the pastor's son to give to children living in the slums of India. Another local Indian pastor requests Memory Books for the children attending his church. In addition, I receive requests from children's homes in Uganda and Kenya.

During the flight home from India, Dr. Kaye asks me if I am interested in conducting research related to the use of the Memory Book. After eight years of placing Memory Books in the hands of children, why wouldn't I be curious about the impact they are making?

With an IRB (International Research Board) approval from University of Portland to conduct a qualitative phenomenological research related to the use of Memory Books by children orphaned in South Africa, Dr. Kaye, Dr. Barb Braband, University of Portland professor and expert in suffering, and I leave for South Africa in March 2012. I do not share my concern for returning to South Africa, yet it dominates my thoughts. This may be the only time I have not wanted to come to Africa. I am committed, though, because of the offer by two very experienced researchers to accompany me and help me uncover the value of a Memory Book. Malcolm and Beverly have agreed to once again host us during our two-week stay while we visit two children's villages where Memory Books have been placed since 2005 and 2006.

After the thirty-two-hour flight, I am ecstatic to see Malcolm when we exit immigration in the beautiful new Durban Airport built for the South Africa-hosted 2010 World Cup. South Africa is literally the furthest from Oregon than anywhere else on earth. If you could draw a line through the globe, you would find South Africa exactly opposite to Oregon. This trip marks my sixth trip to South Africa. Malcolm and Beverly have sold their beautiful opulent home and purchased a smaller Dutch Colonial style home on five acres in Kloof. The home has a beautiful setting under grand trees, but is in desperate need of renovation. I could see why they bought the home; it has the same lovely feel of old world charm centered on family living. With their son Gareth still away at Stellenbosch University in Cape Town and their daughter Alex away at boarding school, there is enough room for the three of us to have our own bedrooms.

After a few days of rest, Kaye, Barb, and I drive to a local church where a beading cooperative of women sell their jewelry, handbags, clothing, and linens. Outside in the shade of the church, chairs are filled with people waiting to be called to fill the need for a housekeeper, landscaper, maintenance man, nanny, or seamstress that day. Church members collect the money made by everyone inside and out, and distribute it equally amongst everyone. I have arranged to take my friends on a tour of Sinikithemba HIV/AIDS Clinic and McCord Hospital. When I enter Sinikitemba clinic I am overcome with emotion as I realize the clinic has created an entire area for the treatment of children. The portable buildings and walls are painted with childlike murals. Children's toys and a play yard are in the center. A staff person tells us about the use of the Memory Books by children when we find hundreds sitting on shelves in an office.

Just before we leave, I see a woman tapping on the window. When she realizes I have seen her she howls and waves her hands. It is a staff person I worked with at Sinikithemba in 2005 during my first trip to South Africa. When we embrace, she simply says, "Can you believe what we've done here? It is because of you, Tamara. It is because of what you taught us." I am reminded of the seed I came to plant many years ago, and am overwhelmed when I realize without my knowledge it produced this beautiful place for children to simply be children. Dr. Holst tells us Sinikithemba HIV/AIDS Clinic is closing except for the children's program. Adults will now be a part of a governmental program set up by Pepfar HIV/AIDS assistance, but the children will still enjoy the child-friendly surroundings created at Sinikithemba clinic. Dr. Holst invites us to dinner at the Oyster Bar in downtown Durban, overlooking the Indian Ocean and endless horizon. A perfect setting for what I dream. Over scrumptious seafood and wine, Dr. Holst asks, 'Tamara, tell me, how is that 'pioneering work' of yours going?"

"I am so glad you asked," I smile. I always love it when I am asked.

Although I have been in contact with the children's villages prior to our coming, this research will require fully outlining the process and obtaining permission from the legal guardian to interview the children about their Memory Books so it is liable to take some persuasive arguments to convince those who are responsible for protecting already vulnerable children. With the passage of time, road improvements, and changes we are lost trying to find a children's village purposely hidden in a sugar cane field at the end of a dirt road. When I see the large tree occupied by Under the Tree women I am relieved to know we have finally found the children's village nearby, merely moments before I am willing to give up.

As we sit down in the office of a newly hired social worker named Karin, I notice the Memory Book Training Manual sitting on her desk. "Oh, yes," she said. "I am very interested in the use of the Memory Book and had hoped to read it before you came." Our conversation seems to come full circle again and again with a sense that Karin feels uncomfortable with the interview process. Dr. Kaye shares her experience with post-abortion interviews, reporting women actually felt they benefitted by sharing their story. She suggests that while we recognize the vulnerability of these children is of highest regard, one of the most important pieces to the preservation of their story is the opportunity to tell their story. The interview process will simply involve looking at a child's Memory Book and having them explain the contents, as we are their witness.

Within minutes we have Karin's approval. We return the next day to interview any children who want to show us their Memory Book. The children's Memory Books are filled with photographs of the child and friends. As each child turns a page, the contents of their own personal Memory Book evoke memories of the event the keepsake or photograph represents. Often, a child wants to revisit particular pages or certain keepsakes. The pondering or remembering appears to be an important part of the interview process for the child. Some of the keepsakes represent relationships the children had with sponsors, one another, or a community member. Sometimes laughter erupts between the child and their peers, but sometimes a child becomes quiet and even tearful as they look at their book. Asked about favorite things, a child will point to a photograph of himself with friends, a field day award, a greeting card from a grannie, or letter from a sponsor.

We experience a similar response when children at another children's village share their personal Memory Books with us. We interviewed a total of thirty children. The most frequent comment regarding the value of having a Memory Book: I want to keep my Memory Book until I am old, or until I die, or forever. When asked if they preferred looking at their personal Memory Book alone or with someone, the majority of children liked looking at it with someone. A young girl sang to us while covering her face after telling us one of her gifts is the ability to sing.

On the long flight home, I had time to think about what we each had experienced. The children's faces, their voices, the emotion of it all etched on my mind. I felt it a privilege to look at a Memory Book with its owner. Inside, I feel sorry I had almost missed the opportunity because of my own fear. I am truly amazed at what we had found: beautiful keepsakes and artifacts of a child's life, preserved for all time.

In the darkness of the airplane cabin and with my mind quiet, I heard a small, yet familiar voice say, *I simply wanted to show you what I've been doing while you've been gone.*

Buoyed by the results of the South Africa research, I decide to return to India with Dr. Kaye and twenty university nursing students in 2013 to continue interviewing children who had Memory Books for two years. With all the necessary protocol in place for conducting valid research, I returned again to India, this time bringing my husband Ron.

Over a period of two weeks, I interview thirty children from three different children's villages and invite the nursing students to help collect data by recording field notes on body language, facial expressions, emotions, even room conditions. These Memory Books appear to be less about storing artifacts and more about written stories. With a translator, each child reads page after page describing in great detail their lives, their families, their favorite school subject, and life as it is now. Sometimes a drawing of their family or of themselves accompanies the written words.

Late one evening after a day of interviews, the room had darkened with only a single bulb of light hanging from the ceiling. Eight young girls are waiting to show us their Memory Books, so we invite all eight to come together. As the first young girl reads from the page about her family, she begins to cry when she reads the words of her mother and father dying. One child after another cries as they read the page describing the deaths of those they love. Each one surrenders into my arms as they sob from deep within. I brush the hair back from the forehead of one young girl and hold her as she cries.

I think to myself what an honor it is to stand in for her mother, to be the physical arms and loving embrace her mother can no longer offer. I sense each young girl's mother somewhere nearby in spirit, longing to hold her child in comfort. When I look up, the translator, tears streaming down his cheeks, simply repeats what was last said, often hesitating as he swallows hard. I wonder if in an attempt to make life happy for children there is no room left for tears or sorrow. I quietly wonder if this may be the first time their tears are accepted and honored. When everyday needs press to the front of any given day, is there time to grieve what once was and still focus on what is with gratitude? There is something more comforting than crying alone in the secrecy of darkness when sadness and grief come—being swaddled in the arms of a loving human being whose compassion brings comfort, if for only a moment.

On the day we leave India, two small girls summon me to come where they are hiding behind a bush. Each bears a beautiful smile. One girl slowly opens her hand to me to reveal a pair of red and clear beaded earrings. "Take them," she said with glistening smile coming from her eyes. "We want you to have them," they whisper. I am overcome to think an orphaned child would offer to give away something she holds dear.

"Are you sure?" I ask. "Yes, please," they shake their heads smiling even broader. "Yes, please." As I reach out to take their precious gift to me, I realize at this moment our stories merge, rewarding each of us with greater meaning and intimacy in the lives we live. This moment, a simple yet profound memory, is indelibly written on each of our hearts forever.

Chapter 25

God Heals Broken Hearts

Waking the morning of the day I would speak at United in Love, a Women of Purpose conference in Nakuru, Kenya, I knew without doubt the Holy Spirit had been speaking to me all night. I woke with clear understanding of what I was to speak about, the format, the words, even analogies as though I had rehearsed meticulously over weeks. It would require my setting aside my agenda and the carefully constructed teaching on Passing on Our Spiritual Heritage for another time. But would I be confident enough to let go of that carefully constructed agenda to make room for God?

With heart thumping and knees wobbling, I walked to the microphone. I wondered if I was crazy for stepping in front of a large crowd without one note. I revealed my dream, joking of rehearsing the dynamic delivery methods and command of the Scriptures and attempting to become a preacher like the previously day's speakers. I said, "It appears it takes a lot longer than one night to become a preacher." Inside, my insecurities of my quiet speaking style rumbled around, attempting to disrupt my train of thought. Then I heard the Lord say, *Why don't you just be yourself?*

"I'm not a preacher, but I am a teacher. I am inviting you to come into my classroom today," I said. "The role of a teacher is to help others unlock the passion for learning and to discover something her students did not previously know."

"What do you know about atmospheric pressure?" Faces around the room looked puzzled as I began. I described the role of atmospheric pressure in changing the weather. "You cannot see atmospheric pressure, but you can see the effects of its presence. When the pressure changes, the wind begins to blow, rushing in cooler or warmer temperatures. The greater the pressure change the greater the wind and change in weather. Small changes may cause leaves to fall from trees, while great atmospheric pressure changes may uproot trees, blow roofs off houses, topple buildings, and even level entire towns. Atmospheric pressure is like the grief that affects us after we lose something. You cannot see grief, but its presence wreaks havoc in our lives. When we lose something dear to us, we grieve the absence. Grief, like a hurricane, produces depression and overwhelming sadness, stomach ailments, headaches, lack of concentration, sleeplessness or sleepiness, lack of motivation, and even anger. Grief can produce these symptoms and more for years following a loss, such as the death of a loved one, or loss of a job, a dream, your independence, or your health. These physical and emotional symptoms are often never associated with the loss because life goes on as time passes. When we lose something dear to us, we are often left alone with our grief and loss because others' lives continue on. Others wonder how long we will be affected by the loss, and often try to distract us with activity or by well meaning phrases intended to 'help us forget'. The truth is we never forget when we have lost something dear to us, or someone we love, or something that changes our lives forever."

Stepping out from behind the podium, I began to walk down the aisle of the church. "I know a young Rwandan boy whose father left his mother," I continued. "His mother could not care for him, so she took him to a local farmer who accepted him to care for his herd of goats. He took the young boy into the fields and left him there," I paused, "for two years. He ate, slept, and lived with the animals. His hair was wild and filled with brambles and bugs. His clothes were tattered, and he was filthy from head to bare toes. When people saw him they were afraid and turned and ran away.

"I know a young Rwandan boy," I continued, "who witnessed the murder and dismemberment of his father, and the rape and killing of his mother and siblings. He was only four years old and hid under a bed. He always felt guilty he did not leave his hiding place to help save his family.

"I know a young Congolese girl who was born crippled and left abandoned by the side of the road where people passing by ignored her.

"I know a baby whose mother died of AIDS. Family members left her wrapped in a blanket next to the gate of an orphanage in South Africa.

Before someone would find her tiny frame she had cried herself hoarse, and was bitten by insects, leaving her pale skin swollen and red.

"I know a man who chose alcohol instead of his job, his wife, and family and now is alone and has lost everything.

"I know an elderly woman who has become so crippled she can no longer walk in her neighborhood visiting people, gathering food, bartering for things she needs.

"I know a South African family whose mother has died leaving the children orphaned and on their own. The children's lives were at risk of contracting the deadly disease that took their mother's life.

"I know young orphaned Indian girls who will be sold into sex slavery if someone does not rescue them from the streets.

"I know a woman whose dearly loved son died, leaving her deeply depressed. Every day she wakes up to the nightmare that has become real.

"I know young Congolese boys who were abducted and taught to murder, rape, and steal as child soldiers.

"I know a young Rwandan girl has lost the hope and dream of becoming educated attending college—because she is an orphan.

"I know a man whose wife has been killed in an automobile accident leaving the man and his children distraught and grief stricken. "

Letting all the stories waft through the air, I stood quietly. The room was quiet. Most eyes were downcast. "I am wondering," I said quietly, "is there anyone in this room who has a similar story?" The words fell gently upon the hush that had filled the room.

Softly and carefully I asked again, "Is there anyone in this room who has lost someone they loved?" I waited a minute without speaking.

"Would you stand?" I asked. "Would you stand and let us know we are not alone with the pain of our loss?" Immediately nearly half the people all over the room stood to their feet, including the entire front row of dignitaries, the local pastor, and local bishop.

I continued, "Is there anyone who has been orphaned?" Dozens stood to their feet. "Is there anyone who was born with an infirmity that has prevented you from achieving your dreams?" Several stood to their feet.

"Has anyone lost their job? Lost a dream? Stand," I said, "and let others see we are not alone." Several more stood while many still stared downward.

"Is there anyone who struggles with alcoholism, drug addiction that has led to losing everything dear to you?' Stand and let others see they are not alone with their losses. Several more people stood to their feet.

"Is there anyone who has simply lost all hope? Stand." I asked once again. I looked around and nearly everyone in the room was standing.

"Look around you," I suggested, "and see you are not alone with your loss. There is someone who knows what it is to lose someone you dearly love. There is someone who knows what it is like to lose a dream, a job, a child, mobility, freedom, even hope.

"You may take your seat," I said. I took a breath, searching my mind for the next thing to say.

"Did you know our bodies are created to heal themselves? Does anyone here have a cut or broken skin?" I roamed the room for an example. "I have a wound on my left temple when a tree branch scratched me while hiking two weeks ago. See?" I pointed to the large scab created by dried blood.

"When the skin is broken, blood rushes to the site, initiating the early stages of healing and rebuilding the skin using the clotting cascade of blood. Blood, with its unique components is designed to knit together fibers within blood to create new skin. Protected by the scab, the broken skin is knitted together by blood itself. Amazing, but that is how God created our bodies to repair broken skin. God knew how fragile our skin was, and created a way to prevent us from losing blood through open wounds, even bleeding to death. Even the scab provides a necessary role in protecting the healing process.

"Has anyone here a broken bone?" Several people raised their hands, and accounts of accidents resulting in broken bones were shared. "When a bone is broken, " I said, "the body brings necessary calcium and minerals to the site of the broken bone, by way of the blood. When the bone is held in place by a cast, the blood transports the necessary components to rebuild the bone completely. Some say, even stronger than the original bone itself.

"Amazing, but that is how God created our broken bones to heal. God knew we needed healthy bones, and so He created a way for our broken bones to heal when carefully supported by a plaster cast. Today, each one of us has acknowledged the losses we have suffered. When someone died, it broke your heart. When a job was lost, or a dream died, it broke your heart. When your health failed, or your addiction took over, or life was turned upside down, or something happened that changed everything forever, you were left with a broken heart.

"Unlike broken skin or bones, broken hearts are difficult to detect from the outside. We often will hide our broken heart from others. We often will deny our broken heart, even to ourselves. There is no way I can tell you have a broken heart, and you cannot tell I have a broken heart simply by looking on the outside."

I took my stethoscope from my bag, and placed it around my neck. "Is there anyone here who would allow me to assess for a broken heart?" I surveyed the quiet room. I looked over to the bishop, who had stood early in the presentation. He admitted to the loss of his dearly beloved wife during his sermon the previous day, but now avoided eye contact with me. Inside I questioned whether I would be violating his dignity by calling him out.

"Bishop?" I shyly asked. "Would you allow me to assess you for a broken heart?" Hesitating for a moment, he then stood, agreeing with a nod of his head. I explained it is very difficult to assess for a broken heart, and placed the stethoscope over his heart. As I mimicked the sound of a beating heart in the microphone, the room filled with laughter. Even the bishop laughed. "That's funny," I suggested. "I do not hear anything unusual, no clanging or banging." The room erupted with laughter, and the bishop laughed out loud.

"Clearly, you have admitted to having a broken heart, but as you can see it is very difficult to detect from the outside." He agreed, smiled, and sat down.

"Anyone else?" I moved to the back of the room where an elderly woman who stood when I had suggested that infirmities kept people from living a full life. When our eyes met, she smiled and painfully stood to her feet again. I placed the stethoscope over her heart. Again, I suggested, the heart did not reveal its brokenness from the outside, but clearly she was broken-hearted over her physical limitations.

Another woman stood and suggested she had a broken heart. Again, the mimicking sound of the heart beating in the microphone brought laughter across the room. She smiled and sat down. "Yes, it is almost impossible to detect a heart that is broken. Like those who stood today, it requires the testimony of the person who has suffered a loss revealing his brokenness." I suggested if everyone knew with certainty that God would heal them at that moment, they would all be on their feet wanting to be assessed for a broken heart, not knowing what God was about to do.

"Do you know God did not forget broken hearts?" I continued reciting that which I had dreamt. "Just like skin, bones, or everything in the body, the very blood that the heart circulates throughout the entire body is essential for the health of the heart itself. The heart uses oxygen-rich blood, directly from the lungs, first before the pumping heart sends it to the other parts of the body. The blood is the vehicle that brings life-producing elements like oxygen and fuel, antibodies against illness and disease, as well as carries away things like carbon dioxide and dead cells that threaten health and wellbeing. The very blood that immerses the heart is not only responsible for the health of the heart, but the entire body. Yes, God did not forget to design healing for our broken hearts and lives. Let us pray and ask God to heal our hearts."

The next day, with an undeniable joy across his face, the bishop jumped to the stage to speak and announced, "While our sister spoke yesterday, God miraculously healed my broken heart of eighteen years, and gave me a heart once again filled with joy. It helped knowing I was not the only one who had suffered loss, but that nearly everyone in this community has lost something or someone."

With each subsequent day of the conference, I witnessed the release of joy and freedom across the faces of all those who were there. The once crippled elderly woman danced down the aisle with more vitality then someone half her age. Every single person in attendance danced and sang with radiating joy and passion. There was no doubt God had touched and healed hearts!

The truth is God always determined it would be blood that brings healing for everything that is broken in our lives. Before we were even created, God made a way for our brokenness to be fully restored by the blood, the life-giving blood His own Son Jesus shed on the cross on our behalf.

This blood carried away all the things that cause death, not carbon dioxide and toxins, but sin, bitterness, and unforgiveness. This blood contained all the elements necessary for life, not oxygen and fuel, but forgiveness, grace, mercy, and the unconditional love of God. This blood heals our brokenness and fills the spaces that are empty in our lives from loss.

Scheduled to speak again, I stand behind the podium of the conference and deliver the original message I brought with me to Kenya titled "Passing on Our Spiritual Heritage." Without warning, two men who had been sitting near the back stand and begin crying, "Pastor, pastor" as they walk toward the front. Both the pastor and bishop meet the men as they make their way forward. The men are red-eyed and stumbling, obviously drunk. I step away from the podium and begin to pray. The pastor and bishop speak to the men in Swahili. With tears streaming down their faces, the men kneel and the pastor and bishop lay hands on their shoulders and begin to pray. When they stand, the pastor announces the men had desperately wanted to accept Jesus as their Savior and simply could not wait. I imagine all heaven's inhabitants celebrating for these two men, and we all begin to shout "Hallelujah!"

Although science attempts to understand the full process of knitting together of skin fibers or creation of new bone, there are aspects of the process that are truly a mystery. And so it is with the healing of your broken heart. I have explained the process, but the healing is truly a mystery of God that requires our simply believing God can heal a broken heart by the blood of Jesus. How God does it is His mystery that is hidden beneath His love for you so endless there is nothing God cannot heal.

Upon arriving home from Kenya, I cry when I received these messages:

"Your comfort and kind words gave me the courage to face my exams and the future. The emptiness, loneliness, and the sadness that had engulfed me since my parents died is no more." – A Kenyan Teenager

"My heart was healed on the day you spoke. My father died when I was but one day old. We lived a hard life of struggle. I will never be the same." – A Kenyan Pastor

Chapter 26

Telling Your Story Matters

While I was a small girl, I loved to swing in the homemade swing my father built in the backyard. Often alone, I kicked and pushed my feet higher and higher as I glided into the air my feet skimming what I thought must be the under side of heaven. I sang to myself, *Somewhere over the rainbow, way up high. Birds fly over the rainbow. Why then, oh why, can't I?* I sensed something out there, but didn't know what until an elderly woman in my neighborhood told me how much God loves me. I felt loved by this woman. There was a peace in that moment I now know to be God himself reaching out to me through someone who cared enough to be a witness to my story.

When I was a lonely, broken child I never dreamt God would one day birth a passion in me to follow Him around the world in search of lonely broken children needing to hear a message of hope. As a mother, I never imagined I could love so many children beyond my own. When I became a nurse, I never imagined I would choose to give up a career to sit close to children as they tell their stories of love and loss. When God captured my heart, through Jesus His Son, everything changed. Instead of comfort and convenience I choose God. Instead of my way, I choose God's way. Instead of accolades, I choose God who chooses me to be His own. Through the eyes of every child I have ever met, I have learned to love the one who peers back at me from life's mirror because I am one of a kind, uniquely and wonderfully made to be His child. Today, I am the woman who wants every child to know they are loved by God.

Telling your story matters because there is only one you.

You are unique and one of a kind. If an ancient Chinese vase, rare blue diamonds, or irreplaceable centuries old violin is valued and considered priceless, imagine your value. You were created as one of a kind. You are priceless, indeed. There will never be another you. There are certainly others who have similar talents, passions, or personalities, but there is no one with exactly what makes you 'you'!

Even when you compare shared experiences others never view life events such as traumatic losses, achievements, or even growing up in the same household from the exact same perspective. A white daisy turns blue in a vase of blue water, but it remains a daisy. Life experiences don't change who God created you to be, they just color your perspective.

Sitting alongside South African children while looking at their personal Memory Books, one by one, it was obvious each one was as unique as the painted handprints that graced the book's front cover. Orphaned and living in a children's village, yet each story was unique.

A young girl wearing sunglasses that cover her entire face except her beautiful smile points to a photograph of herself with her friends when asked, "What is your favorite thing in your Memory Book?' Another points to her School Field Day blue ribbon. A young boy lingers over a page covered with dozens of stick figures he had drawn in pencil. "This is my family," he says. A young girl carefully pulls out a letter tucked inside her Memory Book and begins to read a letter she has addressed to God. "Everyone in my family has died except me and my brother. I am grateful for my life." She looks into my eyes and carefully returns this treasure to its safe place inside her Memory Book.

Each child's life story was told through photographs, drawings, stories, schoolwork and awards, letters and greeting cards, and keepsakes—all capable of helping a child sense I am somebody, after losing so much of what defined their identities.

Telling your story helps grieve losses and promote healing.

When you experience loss, whether a loved one, a dream, your independence or health, innocence, or even a cherished possession like a home, the human response is to mourn on the outside and grieve on the inside. But the external pressures of jobs and other responsibilities, well-meaning people, and our own desire to escape the pain of loss cause us to ignore grief while it exerts its effects inside.

Instead of making room to grieve a loss by taking time to make sense of what has happened and how it will affect our life, we push down the pain and get busy with living. The symptoms of the grief response such as stomach or head ache, lethargy or anger, poor concentration, or risk taking, just to name a few, are often not associated with loss, but are addressed as poor work ethic, rebellion, bad eating habits, or depression. The internal presence of grief is like the atmospheric pressure that creates weather changes. Like atmospheric pressure, you cannot see grief but only its effects on the person; the greater the loss the greater the effects.

Eight young Indian girls sat around the table holding their personal Memory Books on their laps. As each one came and sat in the chair next to me and read the words "died," it seemed as though they welcomed the opportunity to allow the pain inside to escape through tears as the words floated into the air. During a Memory Book training session, a young Indian man explained the need to lead his family bravely after the death of his father. When he looked up, his face was stained by the release of hidden tears. In South Africa, while other children showed their Memory Books, a young girl without a Memory Book held a small toy bear to her chest. When she was handed a personal Memory Book, she laid down the bear and held the Memory Book to her chest. An adolescent South African boy rejected the offer to show his Memory Book, but instead wanted to look at it alone. Some children laughed, some children cried. But they all grieved.

The Memory Book is a valuable tool in the grief process, allowing thoughts and feelings surrounding traumatic events to be recorded and reassessed over time. The journey of grief is not linear or predictable, but circular and is uniquely individual. The destination of healing may take a lifetime.

Telling your story matters because your life story intersects with other life stories.

When we tell our story, we may gain or give greater insight, perspective, and truthfulness to others surrounding traumatic events. Our lives are often deeply impacted by events and losses that occur before we are old enough to fully comprehend the meaning of the event. The retelling or rumination or discussion with others over time and maturity may foster enhanced understanding of the event, and promote grieving of a personal loss.

The children exhibited genuine interest in one another's story by quietly listening, and wanting to look closer, often laughing or smiling at one another's photographs or drawings. They liked to see their own photograph in someone's Memory Book. "This is my family," a young boy said about a photograph of his housemother and children living in the same cottage. When housemothers attended training in the use of the Memory Book, they each stood and told a story of a picture they had drawn of their own personal tragedy or loss. They discovered the gift of simply being a witness to someone's story, and the healing that comes when you discover someone wants to listen or shares a similar story cultivating intimacy in relationships.

Telling your story matters because it promotes resiliency and hope for a future.

The preservation and telling of one's story improves the potential for recovery and healing from traumatic crisis with guidance and support from one or more caring people, a vital factor in achieving resilience.[15] Journaling or the telling of one's story improves the potential for exceeding a sense of recovery and realizing actual growth from an event.[16] Drawings facilitate more effective communication with children, and allow children to convey their thoughts and feelings when words are too difficult or language skills not yet developed.[17]

Throughout the interviews were numerous examples of children remembering those they had lost as well as their new relationships.

Children were able to use their Memory Books to tell their stories, often without words. Numerous children shared stories of themselves in the future by identifying hopes and dreams. Many of the stories were about hobbies, schoolwork, spirituality, and sports, exhibiting evidence of coping mechanisms to help shore up their lives. A teenage South African boy had drawn a picture of himself driving a jeep saying, "I want to be a game ranger one day." Another boy said, "I want to be a soccer player," pointing to a drawing inside his Memory Book.

The children held their Memory Books close. When asked how long they would keep their Memory Book, many exclaimed, "Until I am old!" Many expressed they would treasure them forever. Children's personal Memory Books are stored on shelves in offices and closets for safekeeping. Some are tucked under children's pillows.

"I think the real impact of the Memory Book will be when they look back on them in ten or twenty years, and they have a real memory of their childhood," summarized one care provider about the value of the Memory Book. "They were just excited, I think, to have something that's theirs. So there was a lot of excitement that 'This is my Memory Book' and 'I'm going to look at it.' It gives them time to really reflect and to think because often these children live in the moment. They're playing and they're in the moment and I think it's good for them to think." While these children were remarkably vulnerable in physiological and psychological characteristics, they exhibited and conveyed an aura of hope and strength in the midst of loss.

A young South African boy pointed to a drawing in his Memory Book as we sat together. "That is me," he said. "And that is a bird, and one day the bird and I are going to fly away." What a beautiful story I hope the whole world will hear one day.

Some of the world's greatest leaders and world-changers have lived lives filled with traumatic crises, yet we would have never known if their stories behind their success had not been told. Inspiration comes from knowing someone has endured through crisis and loss, yet lived a life of purpose and passion in spite of it all.

When I think of the stories I have heard from around the world, I am reminded of the tiny alpine flower growing and beautifully blooming high atop Kilimanjaro despite the mighty storms and inhospitable environment it survives. Its creation is not by accident or mistake, but God designed the delicate flower for the purpose of inspiring us all.

Chapter 27

Memory Books for Children

After ten years and the shipment of 25,000 Memory Books to children living in South Africa, Tanzania, Nigeria, Rwanda, The Democratic Republic of the Congo, Uganda, Kenya, India, Thailand, Indonesia, Bangladesh, Haiti, Mexico, and the USA, I have discovered an amazing intersection. Whether an orphaned child or a grieving child trapped inside an adult body, research shows Memory Books are a valuable tool to re-establish a sense of identity, enjoy meaningful relationships with others, and reveal hopes and dreams for a future with purpose after suffering loss and grief.

Anyone involved in Memory Books would likely tell you this: Being involved in the Memory Book outreach to children around the world gives my life purpose, and I am important to God. I am somebody God can use to touch the lives of children grieving some of the life's greatest losses, even though I, too, have endured similar experiences.

Anyone involved in Memory Books would likely say the Memory Book outreach provides an opportunity to enjoy relationships with others and God Himself. Anyone involved in Memory Books would likely tell you being involved provides them opportunity to cope with life's disappointments and devastating losses while using gifts and talents that give to others. Being connected with Memory Books brings both joy and tears, for themselves and for the children served.

Children who have received Memory Books tell me, "I learned I am unique and special to God. I am somebody." When asked to show their favorite thing preserved on its pages, they frequently point to their photo with friends or a letter they've received. After losing everything, children treasure relationships. When I ask children what brings them joy, they point to sports awards, hobbies, and school that provide them an opportunity to discover life can once again be enjoyed. For the children, joy and tears co-exist in their hearts and on their faces.

Ask anyone involved in Memory Books and they would likely tell you being involved in the Memory Book outreach inspires hope rising up from their own darkest moments as they see God using something so simple as a scrapbook to touch a child's life. As I ask children what they hope for, I see that their Memory Books are filled with dreams for a future. When asked, many children say they will keep their Memory Book forever—a priceless treasure.

Dr. Kaye Wilson Anderson, co author of Evaluation of Utilization of Memory Books by Orphaned Children in South Africa research, said, "Tamara, it is exciting to see the desired outcomes to an intervention you introduced. By faith, you simply took one step after another, and look where it has led. Dr. Holst, of McCord Hospital called it 'pioneering work.' I simply call it God's work. "

God created the body to heal itself. The clotting cascade that knits together torn tissue or the import of calcium and minerals to repair a broken bone heals damage when being supported by a bandage or cast. God has not forgotten broken hearts. Damaged hearts are His specialty because He designed them to be healed by His love and the love and support of others.

God loves the children of the world so much He has asked us to take the message to them through a simple scrapbook. God wants children to know He created each one unique and special, and that they are important to Him. God hears all their prayers and will answer every single one. God sees their tears and will mend their broken hearts. God has designed a plan and purpose in the world for each of them. God loves the children of the world so much He wants them to know He will never ever leave them alone. God offers to be Father to the fatherless, to call each His own. This message with a profound purpose is delivered in a simple scrapbook.

Chapter 28

Part of Your Story
Can Be Part of Their Story

Have you suffered the loss of someone you love? Have you suffered the loss of doing something you love? Your health or independence? Have you lost a dream? Or the hope for your future?

What would it mean to discover there is someone who cares? To discover I AM SOMEBODY?

The greatest gift you can give a child is to be a witness to their life with compassion and understanding.

The goal of Memory Books for Children is to gift children with Memory Books and Memory Book Clubs that invite them to tell their story, begin the journey of healing, and discover their special role in God's greater story.

Your purchase of *I Am Somebody* will fund one Memory Book for a child. Any other donation to Memory Books for Children will fund additional Memory Books and supplies for Memory Book Clubs.

Memory Books 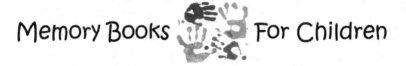 For Children

helping children tell their stories in the midst of loss
www.memorybooks4children.com
P.O. Box 1372
Gresham, Oregon 97030

Epilogue

As you have turned the pages of this story, it is my deepest desire that your own story has begun to emerge. Not for torment, but to bring it into the light. I pray you will find comfort and peace in your brokenness and hour of need, knowing God has been and always is near to the brokenhearted. May the God of miracles touch and heal your heart and life by filling every empty space with His love and satisfy all your deepest longings. This is not the end of the story, but only the beginning as God reveals the purpose for the experiences you have lived on your journey to discover "I am somebody," because He is the Great I AM!

Acknowledgements

Words seem inadequate to acknowledge and thank those who have loved, supported, and guided me, not only when I lived this amazing journey of faith and discovery, but also long before.

Thank you to my adoring husband, Ron, who loved me long before I learned to love myself, and loves God enough to hold me close and to let me go. Thank you for believing, even when I did not. Thank you for showing me how to not fear, but live a life of passion, adventure, and purpose for God.

Thank you to my children and grandchildren for sacrificing your own sense of peace when I have risked following God to faraway places. Thank you for sharing me with the world's children. Thank you for giving to me my richest gift in life—your love.

Thank you to my sister Pamela and brother Gordon, and my departed sister Denyce, for helping me recognize while living under the same roof that each of our stories is unique. Thank you to my dear friend, Debbie L; your love and friendship gave me courage to look at the brokenness and grieve.

Thank you to my editor, Linda D, for guidance and assurance especially in the early days and months of writing this book, and for the countless hours editing and for all the hours of personal reflection over coffee that affirmed the universal meaning of the story. Thank you to Stacy B, Holly

F, Holly H, Elaine E, Anita and Bruce P, Dr. Holst, Leslie N, and Barb for proofreading. Thank you Stacie B for the beautiful book cover design and using your creative gifts that helped get this book print ready.

Thank you to the hundreds of individuals who give of their time, resources, and support to purchase, assemble, and ship Memory Books, art supplies, gifts, and write letters to children living with loss around the world. Thank you to Holly F, Stacy, Terri, Andrea, Lynette, Elaine, Linda, and Anne for serving and directing this global outreach as Memory Books Advisory Team.

Thank you to Malcolm and Beverly S and Dr. Helga Holst, South Africa; I & S, Nigeria; Bruce and Anita P, The DR of the Congo; E, Rwanda; Innocent, Tanzania; D, Kenya; S and S, India; B, Indonesia; and Dr. O. Virginia Phillips, USA, for serving on the International Advisory Team for Memory Books.

Thank you to Jon Sittko, Clean Fun Promotions Inc., for generously donating the resources, staff, and expertise to design and create, import, store, and ship Memory Books for Children. And thank you to Bethany T for communicating this global outreach so beautifully on the web, newsletter and resource initiative.

Thank you to Kaye and Barb for your expertise and dedication to research related to the use and value of a Memory Book, and the courage to travel to the ends of the earth.

And I want to thank you, the reader. Thank you for responding to your heart, to pick up this book and read it. Your story has now merged with a child's somewhere in the world, because with this book purchase a child will be gifted with a Memory Book to preserve and tell his or her story. And this could just be the beginning of writing a beautiful and meaningful ending to your own story.

Endnotes

1. Maxine Harris, *The Loss That Is Forever: The Lifelong Impact of the Early Death of a Mother or Father* (Plume, 1996).

2. T. Pakenham, *The Boer War*, (New York: Random House, 1979), xiii.

3. L. Cluver, F. Garner, & D. Operario (2009). "Poverty and psychological health among AIDS-orphaned children in Cape Town, South Africa" AIDS Care, 21: 732-741.

4. McCord Hospital, Durban South Africa. PMTCT stats, 2004.

5. Donna Schuurman, *Never the Same: Coming to Terms with the Death of a Parent* (New York: St. Martin's Press, 2003), 109.

6. A. Wolfelt, *Helping Children Cope with Grief* (Routledge, 1983).

7. Donna Schuurman, *Never the Same: Coming to Terms with the Death of a Parent* (New York: St. Martin's Press, 2003).

8. Ibid. 109.

9. "Nkosi Sikelel' iAfrika" ("Lord Bless Africa" in Xhosa), was originally composed as a hymn in 1897 by Enoch Sontonga, a teacher at a Methodist mission school in Johannesburg, to the tune 'Aberystwyth' by Joseph Parry. The song is currently the national anthem of Tanzania, Zambia and since 1994, a portion of the national anthem of South Africa. http://en.wikipedia.org/wiki/National_anthem_of_South_Africa

10. Oswald Chambers, *My Utmost for His Highest.*

11. Oswald Chambers, *My Utmost for His Highest.* 130.

12. S.D. Price, *1001 Smartest Things Ever Said*. (Guilford, CT: The Lyons Press, 2005)168.

13. The mission of The Dougy Center is to provide support in a safe place where children, teens, young adults and their families grieving a death can share their experiences. The Dougy Center, the first center in the United States to provide peer support groups for grieving children, was founded in 1982, in Portland, Oregon. dougy.org.

14. Michael W. Smith, Agnus Dei, Reunion Records, 2001.

15. K.M. Kirwin & V. Harmin (2005). "Decreasing the risk of complicated bereavement and future psychiatric disorders in children." Journal of Child & Adolescent Psychiatric Nursing, 18(1) 62-78.

16. R.G. Tedeschi & L.G. Calhoun (2004). "Posttraumatic growth: Conceptual foundations and empirical evidence." Psychological Inquiry. 15(1), 1-18.

17. P.T. Clements, K.M. Benasutti, & G.C. Henry (2001). "Drawings from experience: Using drawings to facilitate communication." Journal of Psychological Nursing & Mental Health Services, 39(12) 12-30.